Gerald Perlman, PhD
Jack Drescher, MD
Editors

A Gay Man's Guide
to Prostate Cancer

A Gay Man's Guide to Prostate Cancer has been co-published simultaneously as *Journal of Gay & Lesbian Psychotherapy*, Volume 9, Numbers 1/2 2005.

More pre-publication
REVIEWS, COMMENTARIES, EVALUATIONS . . .

"**A**N INVALUABLE HANDBOOK for gay men, their partners, their psychotherapists, and their urologists. . . . Just the right balance of up-to-date medical information, analyses of the pros and cons of current treatment options, exploration of the unique psychological issues prostate cancer poses to sexually active gay men (whether coupled or single), and firsthand accounts by cancer survivors. These men write with candor, courage, and, yes, humor. My partner, who was diagnosed last year, and I could barely put the book down. Bravo!"

Gil Tunnell, PhD
Adjunct Assistant Professor
of Psychology and Education
Teachers College, Columbia University
Co-author of
Couples Therapy with Gay Men

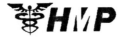

The Haworth Medical Press®
An Imprint of The Haworth Press, Inc.

A Gay Man's Guide
to Prostate Cancer

A Gay Man's Guide to Prostate Cancer has been co-published simultaneously as *Journal of Gay & Lesbian Psychotherapy*, Volume 9, Numbers 1/2 2005.

The *Journal of Gay & Lesbian Psychotherapy* Monographic "Separates"

Below is a list of "separates," which in serials librarianship means a special issue simultaneously published as a special journal issue or double-issue *and* as a "separate" hardbound monograph. (This is a format which we also call a "DocuSerial.")

"Separates" are published because specialized libraries or professionals may wish to purchase a specific thematic issue by itself in a format which can be separately cataloged and shelved, as opposed to purchasing the journal on an on-going basis. Faculty members may also more easily consider a "separate" for classroom adoption.

"Separates" are carefully classified separately with the major book jobbers so that the journal tie-in can be noted on new book order slips to avoid duplicate purchasing.

You may wish to visit Haworth's website at . . .

http://www.HaworthPress.com

. . . to search our online catalog for complete tables of contents of these separates and related publications.

You may also call 1-800-HAWORTH (outside US/Canada: 607-722-5857), or Fax: 1-800-895-0582 (outside US/Canada: 607-771-0012), or e-mail at:

docdelivery@haworthpress.com

A Gay Man's Guide to Prostate Cancer, edited by Gerald Perlman, PhD, and Jack Drescher, MD (Vol. 9, No. 1/2, 2005). *"EXCELLENT. . . . HIGHLY RECOMMENDED. Patients reading this book will find themselves here, and professionals will learn what they need to help their patients as they struggle with these emotional topics." (Donald Johannessen, MD, Clinical Assistant Professor of Psychiatry, NYU School of Medicine)*

Handbook of LGBT Issues in Community Mental Health, edited by Ronald E. Hellman, PhD, and Jack Drescher, MD (Vol. 8, No. 3/4, 2004). *"COMPREHENSIVE . . . Richly strewn with data, useful addresses of voluntary and other organizations, and case histories." (Michael King, MD, PhD, Professor of Primary Care Psychiatry, Royal Free and University College Medical School, London)*

Transgender Subjectivities: A Clinician's Guide, edited by Ubaldo Leli, MD, and Jack Drescher, MD (Vol. 8, No. 1/2, 2004). *"INDISPENSABLE for diagnosticians and therapists dealing with gender dysphoria, important for researchers, and a direct source of help for all individuals suffering from painful uncertainties regarding their sexual identity." (Otto F. Kernberg, MD, Director, Personality Disorders Institute, Weill Medical College of Cornell University)*

The Mental Health Professions and Homosexuality: International Perspectives, edited by Vittorio Lingiardi, MD, and Jack Drescher, MD (Vol. 7, No. 1/2, 2003). *"PROVIDES A WORLDWIDE PERSPECTIVE that illuminates the psychiatric, psychoanalytic, and mental health professions' understanding and treatment of both lay and professional sexual minorities." (Bob Barrett, PhD, Professor and Counseling Program Coordinator, University of North Carolina at Charlotte)*

Sexual Conversion Therapy: Ethical, Clinical, and Research Perspectives, edited by Ariel Shidlo, PhD, Michael Schroeder, PsyD, and Jack Drescher, MD (Vol. 5, No. 3/4, 2001). *"THIS IS AN IMPORTANT BOOK. . . . AN INVALUABLE RESOURCES FOR MENTAL HEALTH PROVIDERS AND POLICYMAKERS. This book gives voice to those men and women who have experienced painful, degrading, and unsuccessful conversion therapy and survived. The ethics and misuses of conversion therapy practice are well documented, as are the harmful effects." (Joyce Hunter, DSW, Research Scientist, HIV Center for Clinical & Behavioral Studies, New York State Psychiatric Institute/Columbia University, New York City)*

Gay and Lesbian Parenting, edited by Deborah F. Glazer, PhD, and Jack Drescher, MD (Vol. 4, No. 3/4, 2001). *Richly textured, probing. These papers accomplish a rare feat: they explore in a candid, psychologically sophisticated, yet highly readable fashion how parenthood impacts lesbian and gay identity and how these identities affect the experience of parenting. Wonderfully informative. (Martin Stephen Frommer, PhD, Faculty/Supervisor, The Institute for Contemporary Psychotherapy, New York City).*

Addictions in the Gay and Lesbian Community, edited by Jeffrey R. Guss, MD, and Jack Drescher, MD (Vol. 3, No. 3/4, 2000). *Explores the unique clinical considerations involved in addiction treatment for gay men and lesbians, groups that reportedly use and abuse alcohol and substances at higher rates than the general population.*

A Gay Man's Guide to Prostate Cancer

Gerald Perlman, PhD
Jack Drescher, MD
Editors

A Gay Man's Guide to Prostate Cancer has been co-published simultaneously as *Journal of Gay & Lesbian Psychotherapy*, Volume 9, Numbers 1/2 2005.

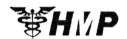

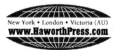

The Haworth Medical Press®
Harrington Park Press®
Imprints of The Haworth Press, Inc.

New York • London • Victoria (AU)
www.HaworthPress.com

Published by

The Haworth Medical Press®, 10 Alice Street, Binghamton, NY 13904-1580 USA

The Haworth Medical Press® is an imprint of The Haworth Press, Inc., 10 Alice Street, Binghamton, NY 13904-1580 USA.

A Gay Man's Guide to Prostate Cancer has been co-published simultaneously as *Journal of Gay & Lesbian Psychotherapy*, Volume 9, Numbers 1/2 2005.

The development, preparation, and publication of this work has been undertaken with great care. However, the publisher, employees, editors, and agents of The Haworth Press and all imprints of The Haworth Press, Inc., including The Haworth Medical Press® and Pharmaceutical Products Press®, are not responsible for any errors contained herein or for consequences that may ensue from use of materials or information contained in this work. Opinions expressed by the author(s) are not necessarily those of The Haworth Press, Inc. With regard to case studies, identities and circumstances of individuals discussed herein have been changed to protect confidentiality. Any resemblance to actual persons, living or dead, is entirely coincidental.

Cover design by Lora Wiggins

Library of Congress Cataloging-in-Publication Data

A gay man's guide to prostate cancer / Gerald Perlman, Jack Drescher, editors.
    p. ; cm.
    "Co-published simultaneously as Journal of gay & lesbian psychotherapy, Volume 9, Numbers 1/2, 2005"
    Includes bibliographical references and index.
    ISBN-10: 1-56023-552-7 (hard cover : alk. paper)
    ISBN-10: 1-56023-553-5 (soft cover : alk. paper)
    ISBN-13: 978-1-56023-552-1 (hard cover : alk. paper)
    ISBN-13: 978-1-56023-553-8 (soft cover : alk. paper)
    1. Prostate–Cancer. 2. Prostate–Cancer–Psychological aspects. 3. Prostate–Cancer–Patients–Mental health. 4. Gay men–Diseases. 5. Gay men–Mental health. I. Perlman, Gerald. II. Drescher, Jack, 1951-. III. Journal of gay & lesbian psychotherapy.
    [DNLM: 1. Prostatic Neoplasms–psychology. 2. Prostatic Neoplasms–rehabilitation. 3. Homosexuality, Male. 4. Life Style. W1 JO663M v. 9 no. 1/2 2005 / WJ 752 G285 2004]
RC280.P7G39 2004
616.99'463'0086642–dc22
                                     2004022875

Indexing, Abstracting & Website/Internet Coverage

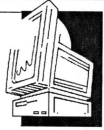

This section provides you with a list of major indexing & abstracting services and other tools for bibliographic access. That is to say, each service began covering this periodical during the year noted in the right column. Most Websites which are listed below have indicated that they will either post, disseminate, compile, archive, cite or alert their own Website users with research-based content from this work. (This list is as current as the copyright date of this publication.)

Abstracting, Website/Indexing Coverage . . . . Year When Coverage Began

- *Abstracts in Anthropology* 1991
- *Academic Index (on-line)* 1992
- *Academic Search Elite (EBSCO)* 1998
- *Academic Search Premier (EBSCO)* 2001
- *Business Source Corporate: coverage of nearly 3,350 quality magazines and journals; designed to meet the diverse information needs of corporations; EBSCO Publishing <http://www.epnet.com/corporate/bsourcecorp.asp>* 1998
- *Contemporary Women's Issues* 1998
- *EBSCOhost Electronic Journals Service (EJS) <http://ejournals.ebsco.com>* 2004
- *e-psyche, LLC <http://www.e-psyche.net>* 2001
- *Expanded Academic ASAP <http://www.galegroup.com>* 1993
- *Expanded Academic ASAP–International <http://www.galegroup.com>* 1993
- *Expanded Academic Index* 1995
- *Family Index Database <http://www.familyscholar.com>* 2003
- *Family Violence & Sexual Assault Bulletin* 1992
- *GenderWatch <http://www.slinfo.com>* 1999

(continued)

(continued)

Special Bibliographic Notes related to special journal issues (separates) and indexing/abstracting:

- indexing/abstracting services in this list will also cover material in any "separate" that is co-published simultaneously with Haworth's special thematic journal issue or DocuSerial. Indexing/abstracting usually covers material at the article/chapter level.
- monographic co-editions are intended for either non-subscribers or libraries which intend to purchase a second copy for their circulating collections.
- monographic co-editions are reported to all jobbers/wholesalers/approval plans. The source journal is listed as the "series" to assist the prevention of duplicate purchasing in the same manner utilized for books-in-series.
- to facilitate user/access services all indexing/abstracting services are encouraged to utilize the co-indexing entry note indicated at the bottom of the first page of each article/chapter/contribution.
- this is intended to assist a library user of any reference tool (whether print, electronic, online, or CD-ROM) to locate the monographic version if the library has purchased this version but not a subscription to the source journal.
- individual articles/chapters in any Haworth publication are also available through the Haworth Document Delivery Service (HDDS).

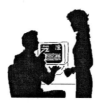

Dedication

The men who have contributed their personal stories to this monograph issue are a self-selected group who are not representative of all gay men with prostate cancer. Nevertheless, they do represent a diverse range of gay men in terms of age, socio-economic status, ethnicity, race, relationship status, treatment choices, and HIV/AIDS status. Each man has used his narrative to open himself up and inform the reader of the unique and universal ways in which he has experienced the diagnosis and treatment of prostate cancer as a gay man. In an informal survey, I asked the men with whom I was working at the time how and in what direction their lives had changed after being diagnosed and/or treated for prostate caner. Over 90% of them replied that after going through the anxieties and depression that frequently accompany such diagnoses and treatment outcomes, their lives had indeed changed and mostly in a positive direction.

Working with men who have been daring enough to share their personal experiences–including those who chose not to write–has been an ongoing source of admiration and joy to me. I am struck by the incredible honesty and courage displayed in these pages. That we can laugh at ourselves, overcome powerful impediments to life as we knew it prior to prostate cancer, and that we can tease one another and just be gay is a remarkable thing.

I want to thank the professionals who contributed to this volume. They struggle every day to diagnose, treat, and understand the uniqueness of each gay man facing prostate cancer.

The Lakota Sioux say that when nature gives one a burden, one is also given a gift. The contributors to this volume have given meaning to that saying. Their courage, self-reflection, and openness are gifts they now give to the reader. So it is to them and the professionals that work with them that I dedicate this volume.

I also dedicate this work to my life partner, David Trachtenberg, who was with me every step of the way; from diagnosis, to treatment, to side effects. He listened to my anxieties, empathized with my depressions, gave me his shoulder to cry on, and helped me celebrate the joys.

Gerald Perlman
May 2004

A Gay Man's Guide
to Prostate Cancer

CONTENTS

ABOUT THE EDITORS

Gerald Perlman, PhD, has been Supervisor of Psychotherapy at Fordham and Yeshiva Universities, and at The City University of New York as well as at The William Alanson White Institute where he received his psychoanalytic training. Dr. Perlman has written numerous articles on the practice of psychotherapy and the mental health issues of gay men. He is Former Director of the Psychology Internship Program at Manhattan Psychiatric Center in NYC. He is also Former President of the New York Association of Gay and Lesbian Psychologists. In his private practice in NYC, he specializes in individual, couples and group treatment. In recent years, he has begun working with gay men with prostate cancer, leading a group of gay men with prostate cancer for Malecare, a not-for-profit self-help organization specifically focusing on gay men with the disease.

Jack Drescher, MD, is a Fellow, Training and Supervising Analyst at the William Alanson White Psychoanalytic Institute. He is Former President of the New York County District Branch, American Psychiatric Association and Chair of the Committee on GLB Concerns of the APA. Author of *Psychoanalytic Therapy and the Gay Man* (1998, The Analytic Press), and Editor-in-Chief of the *JGLP*, Dr. Drescher is in private practice in New York City.

Introduction:
What Gay Men
(and Those Near and Dear to Them)
Need to Know About Prostate Cancer

There was a time, not too long ago, when having cancer was considered so shameful that those individuals diagnosed were treated by others–and regarded themselves–as social pariahs. Fortunately, much has changed. For example, today one finds numerous popular articles and books written about prostate cancer. Prominent figures from politics, sports, the military and entertainment–Rudy Giuliani, Joe Torre, Norman Schwartzkopf, Andy Grove, and Harry Belafonte to name a few–have gone public with their personal stories of coping with prostate cancer. All this is good news, as celebrity stories have brought prostate cancer out of its closet of shame, stigma, and ignorance and into the open daylight. In this way, those men who are affected can get appropriate diagnosis, treatment, and support.

There are some disturbing statistics. Most people probably do not know that prostate cancer is the second leading cause of cancer deaths in men, causing almost 30,000 deaths each year. A man has a one in six chance of developing invasive prostate cancer in his lifetime. It is estimated that approximately 230,900 new cases will be diagnosed in 2004. Nor is it just an older person's disease–the age range of those diagnosed spans from men in their early 30s through those in their 90s.[1,2] In the last decade, medicine has advanced considerably in diagnosing and treating

[Haworth co-indexing entry note]: "Introduction: What Gay Men (and Those Near and Dear to Them) Need to Know About Prostate Cancer." Perlman, Gerald, and Jack Drescher. Co-published simultaneously in *Journal of Gay & Lesbian Psychotherapy* (The Haworth Medical Press, an imprint of The Haworth Press, Inc.) Vol. 9, No. 1/2, 2005, pp. 1-7; and: *A Gay Man's Guide to Prostate Cancer* (ed: Gerald Perlman, and Jack Drescher) The Haworth Medical Press, an imprint of The Haworth Press, Inc., 2005, pp. 1-7. Single or multiple copies of this article are available for a fee from The Haworth Document Delivery Service [1-800-HAWORTH, 9:00 a.m. - 5:00 p.m. (EST). E-mail address: docdelivery@haworthpress.com].

Digital Object Identifier: 10.1300/J236v09n01_01

prostate cancer, although what constitutes the best approach to treatment is controversial.

Despite these alarming statistics and the advantages of early detection, most men either know very little about prostate cancer or they choose *not* to know about it–often until it is too late. This selective inattention is entirely comprehensible. The historical legacy of stigmatizing cancer keeps the subject, even discussions about preventing it, out of everyday awareness.

Among gay men, the subject of prostate cancer is further complicated by the intersecting stigmata of both cancer and homosexuality. Most people do not want to talk about prostate cancer and most straight people do not want to talk about homosexuality. It is therefore not surprising that the overwhelming majority of personal and professional publications about prostate cancer are written by, for and about heterosexual men and their female partners. If prostate cancer, in general, is off most people's radar screen, then gay men with prostate cancer are a truly invisible species.

An invisible clinical population is a troublesome fact, given that clinical experience has shown that most men–gay or straight–are traumatized upon being told they have prostate cancer. Even before the shock of diagnosis abates, every man is confronted with the task of finding the right doctor(s), choosing the right treatment(s), and inevitably dealing with the unwelcome side effects caused by those treatments. These facts require that the man with prostate cancer be patient, informed, persistent, and courageous. It also requires, in the opinion of both the lay and professional contributors to this volume, that he be able to find emotional and psychological support from his partner, his friends, and his doctors. Toward that end, this monograph issue of the *Journal of Gay & Lesbian Psychotherapy* aims to address and shed light upon the needs of that invisible population of gay men (and their partners) confronting prostate cancer.

This monograph issue is aimed not only at the mental health professionals who read the *JGLP* and who may treat gay men with prostate cancer, it is for the patients themselves. It is also intended to be helpful to the partners, family members, support systems and physicians of men with prostate cancer.

The first section addresses prostate cancer from the perspective of health and mental health professionals. The second section consists of papers written from a personal point of view: articles by gay men of diverse ages, races, and ethnicities describing their own experiences with prostate cancer. The final section is a glossary of technical terms.

Vincent Santillo and Frank Lowe, MD, begin the professional section of papers with "Prostate Cancer and the Gay Male." They discuss the basics of prostate cancer with an overview of the causes, diagnosis, screening guidelines and treatments for prostate cancer. They highlight issues of particular concern to gay men, including the potential effect of testosterone supplements, HIV status, anal sex and its impact on PSA testing, and the potential change in sexual response during anal sex resulting from the removal of the prostate. They explore issues of doctor-patient communication as they specifically relate to the gay prostate cancer patient.

Among health professionals, the diagnosis and treatment of prostate cancer often raises more questions than it answers. Consequently, Santillo and Lowe describe a different treatment bias than does David Cornell in "A Gay Urologist's Changing Views on Prostate Cancer." Dr. Cornell traces the history of prostate cancer diagnosis and treatment through the 1980s and '90s to the present. He describes some of the unique concerns that gay men have when consulting with a urologist and making treatment decisions. He also writes about the need for and his development of a gay prostate cancer website. Dr. Cornell argues for the aggressive treatment of prostate cancer, taking into account the need to be aware of lifestyle issues.

In "The Ups and Downs of Gay Sex After Prostate Cancer Treatment," Steven Goldstone, MD, addresses practical questions regarding gay sex after a man has been treated for prostate cancer. He also addresses some of the concerns of the partners of gay man with prostate cancer. Dr. Goldstone offers the reader a practical and matter of fact primer of what may happen during and what to do after prostate cancer treatment.

In "Psychotherapy with Gay Prostate Cancer Patients," Darryl Mitteldorf, LCSW, uses examples from his own practice to highlight psychological issues that surface in individual psychotherapy with gay men diagnosed and treated for prostate cancer. Many of his patients report symptoms of both depression and anxiety. Mitteldorf sees the goal of psychotherapy as reducing the psychological symptoms that result from internalizing the diagnosis and undergoing physical treatment. He warns that as gay men navigate the heterosexually biased world of prostate cancer treatment, they must also confront potential problems of stigmatization, including scarring, ejaculation and erectile dysfunction, and HIV/AIDS envy.

The last professional paper is Gerald Perlman, PhD's, "Prostate Cancer, The Group, and Me." However, it is both a professional and personal contribution. Dr. Perlman writes of his own journey as a gay man dealing with his own prostate cancer that led to his becoming a facilitator of a support group for other gay men with the same disease. He describes the dynamics and concerns of gay men with prostate cancer within the context of a self-help group. Among the topics covered in such groups are gay identities, sexual behaviors and attitudes, feelings of helplessness, anger and loss, HIV/AIDS considerations, partner issues and adaptation.

The second section of personal accounts begins with Roberto Martinez's, "Prostate Cancer and Sex." Martinez, a self-described "sexually active Latino gay man," tells of how the surgical removal of his prostate gland affected his thoughts, feelings, attitudes and activities about sexuality in general. He also speaks more specifically about how the physical changes he experienced engendered emotional changes in his own struggles with sex and masturbation.

Lidell Jackson's "Surviving Yet Another Challenge," also talks about prostate cancer's challenge to his sexuality. Jackson, a self-proclaimed sex-positive gay man, compares the challenge of prostate cancer to the struggle he went through when he seroconverted. As a man of color, Jackson feels particularly strong about alerting his Black brothers to their increased risk of developing prostate cancer.

Jerry Harris had his radical prostatectomy many years prior to the other contributors. In, "Living with Prostate Cancer: One Gay Man's Experience," he tells of his difficulties with the medical community and of his struggle with sexual dysfunction following his surgery. Having looked in vain for support, he describes the formation of his own gay mens' prostate cancer support group. Harris, finally, tells of finding a rainbow at the end of his long struggle.

In "Identity and Prostate Cancer: Comments on a Messy Life," the pseudonymous "Mark Miller" laments what he calls "the devastation" to his sense of self and body image following a radical prostatectomy. He remarks on his own fears of being unacceptable and unappealing in a gay community that he views as being consumed with youth and beauty. In contrast, prominent psychiatrist and psychoanalyst Bert Schaffner, MD, describes how dealing with "Prostate Cancer at Age 84" did not alter his sexual identity. Dr. Schaffner writes that he feels as gay as ever, and in a way feels freer to be more related and affectionate.

In "Together with Prostate Cancer," Robert Parkin and his partner Howard Girven present their particular experience as an older gay couple confronting prostate cancer. Theirs is a unique tale of their respective experiences seeking treatment for their prostate cancers during overlapping times at Loma Linda University Medical Center. They discuss what it was like being gay in that setting and how their sex life has evolved following treatment.

The impact on couples is taken up further by Greg Higgins in "A Gay Man and His Partner Face Prostate Cancer Together." Higgins writes about his experience with the medical profession and the importance of being proactive about one's treatment as well as the need to look for support. He devotes a good portion of his paper to the effect his cancer has had on his relationship of 10 years to a man more than 20 years his junior.

Those who think prostate cancer is just an older man's disease will be startled to read Vincent Santillo's "Prostate Cancer Diagnosis and Treatment of a 33-Year-Old Gay Man." Santillo takes the reader on a personally revealing journey of his struggle with prostate cancer, how it changed him and how it affected his relationship of 12 years.

This issue concludes with Dr. Perlman's glossary of technical terms. Hopefully it will serve as a reference guide and resource for gay men, their partners and family members who are coping with prostate cancer.

The field of prostate cancer is constantly changing. New information is being published daily; views on diagnosis and treatment may vary according to the practitioner/researcher. Statistics, by their very nature, are open to varying interpretations. And each man's experience is unique to him. The goal of this volume is to increase people's knowledge base as they make medical choices. As with any such medical and psychological events, the authors and editors recommend that men with prostate cancer make all their medical choices in consultation with a qualified physician that they trust.

For those interested in obtaining more information, there are a great number of resources available regarding prostate cancer in general. These resources include books, websites, and support groups. The American Foundation for Urologic Disease (AFUD) publishes a Resource Guide for Prostate Cancer. The AFUD may be contacted on the Internet at *www.afud.org*; by phone at (410) 468-1800; or by mail at 1128 North Charles Street, Baltimore, MD 21201-5559.

Although available to the general population of men with prostate cancer as well as those with penile, testicular, and breast cancer, Malecare is the only self-help organization of which we are aware that is particularly responsive to gay men with prostate cancer. With branches across the United States and in several foreign countries, Malecare may be contacted on the Internet at *www.malecare.com/*.

Gerald Perlman, PhD
Jack Drescher, MD

NOTES

1. American Cancer Society (2004), *Cancer Facts & Figures 2004*.
2. Lewis, J. (2003), The PSA test. *The Prostate Cancer Exchange*, 29:3-5 (Sept/Oct).

The Prostate Gland

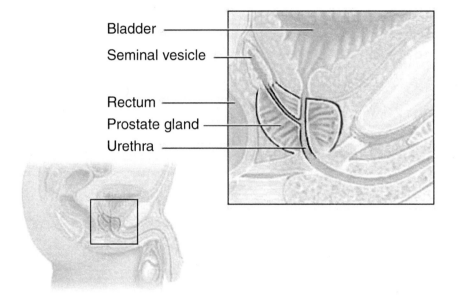

Bladder

Seminal vesicle

Rectum

Prostate gland

Urethra

PROFESSIONAL PERSPECTIVE

Prostate Cancer and the Gay Male

Vincent M. Santillo
Franklin C. Lowe, MD, MPH, FACS

SUMMARY. This is an overview of the causes, screening guidelines and treatments for prostate cancer. The paper also highlights issues of particular concern to gay men including the potential effect of testosterone supplements, HIV status, anal sex and its impact on PSA testing, and the potential change in sexual response during anal sex resulting from the removal of the prostate. Issues of doctor-patient communication as they specifically relate to the gay prostate cancer patient are explored. *[Article copies available for a fee from The Haworth Document Delivery Service: 1-800-HAWORTH. E-mail address: <docdelivery@haworthpress.com> Website: <http://www.HaworthPress.com> © 2005 by The Haworth Press, Inc. All rights reserved.]*

Vincent M. Santillo holds a BS in Economics from the University of Pennsylvania, and an MBA from Columbia University. He is currently enrolled in the Post-baccalaureate Premedical Program at Columbia University.

Franklin C. Lowe is Professor of Clinical Urology, St Luke's/Roosevelt Hospital; Professor of Clinical Urology, Columbia University College of Physicians and Surgeons.

[Haworth co-indexing entry note]: "Prostate Cancer and the Gay Male." Santillo, Vincent M., and Franklin C. Lowe. Co-published simultaneously in *Journal of Gay & Lesbian Psychotherapy* (The Haworth Medical Press, an imprint of The Haworth Press, Inc.) Vol. 9, No. 1/2, 2005, pp. 9-27; and: *A Gay Man's Guide to Prostate Cancer* (ed: Gerald Perlman, and Jack Drescher) The Haworth Medical Press, an imprint of The Haworth Press, Inc., 2005, pp. 9-27. Single or multiple copies of this article are available for a fee from The Haworth Document Delivery Service [1-800-HAWORTH, 9:00 a.m. - 5:00 p.m. (EST). E-mail address: docdelivery@haworthpress.com].

KEYWORDS. AIDS, anabolic steroids, anal sex, cancer, diet, erectile dysfunction, finasteride, gay, gay couples, gay relationships, HIV, homosexuality, impotence, incontinence, informed consent, prostate, prostatectomy, PSA testing, testosterone

INTRODUCTION

Prostate cancer is the second leading cause of cancer death in men, the first being lung cancer. The American Cancer Society anticipated that in 2004, almost 231,000 men in the Unites States would be diagnosed with prostate cancer, and that 29,900 of these men would die of the disease. This represents an increase in the diagnosis of prostate cancer from 220,900 men in 2003, and an increase from the estimate of 189,000 men diagnosed in 2002. The dramatic increase in prostate cancer diagnoses has been due to increased screening for the disease. While the screening has uncovered more and more cases, the increased monitoring has allowed for earlier diagnosis in men with no symptoms of the disease. This in turn has improved the treatment outcomes. In the last 20 years, the five-year survival rate for all stages of prostate cancer has increased from 67% to 97% and the ten-year and fifteen-year survival rates are 79% and 57%, respectively, according to the most recent data (American Cancer Society, 2003; Jemal et al., 2002).

While gay men do not, on the surface, appear to have any specific issues with prostate cancer as compared to heterosexual men, this is not necessarily true. Men have a 17% probability of being diagnosed with prostate cancer in their lifetimes (American Cancer Society, 2003). For a gay couple that means that there is a 28% chance that one partner will be diagnosed with prostate cancer over their lifetime and a 3% chance that both partners will be diagnosed.

Among the several potential issues that gay men and their medical providers need to be aware of are:

- The use of testosterone and other anabolic steroids, whether prescribed for AIDS patients or as a performance enhancer.
- The use of finasteride (Propecia) for hair-loss.
- HIV status and its influence on treatment options.
- Anal sex and its effect on prostate-specific antigen (PSA) tests.
- The effect of poor doctor-patient communication on treatment due to real or perceived issues regarding the patient's sexuality and sexual orientation.

- Post-treatment issues of physical changes and their affects on sexuality and specifically the reduction of sensation during receptive anal intercourse.

RISK FACTORS IN PROSTATE CANCER

While the specific causes of prostate cancer are unknown, there is considerable evidence that both genetics and environment play a role in the evolution of the disease (Reiter, 2002). Risk factors include family history, racial origin, and dietary factors. In addition, several studies have investigated the impact of cigarette smoking and infectious agents and have deemed both factors to have a limited impact on the initiation of the disease (Pienta, 1993). There is some suggestion that positive HIV status may increase the risk of prostate cancer (Crum et al., 2002).

Familial Influences

A number of studies have demonstrated familial clustering of prostate cancer, suggesting that some prostate cancers may be inherited, estimated at 10% of total prostate cancer cases. Men with one first-degree relative (father or brother) with prostate cancer have two times the risk of men who have no relatives with the disease. Men with two or three affected first-degree relatives have a five to eleven-times increased risk, respectively (Reiter and deKernion, 2002; Steinberg et al., 1990). The Johns Hopkins Criteria were developed to help identify families that have a high risk of prostate cancer. According to the Criteria, a family has a high risk if either: (1) prostate cancer has occurred in three or more first-degree relatives; (2) prostate cancer has occurred in three successive generations of either maternal or paternal lineages; or (3) two relatives have been affected at earlier than age fifty-five (Zeegers et al., 2003). According to these authors, "Men with a positive family history of disease constitute an easily identifiable high-risk group that could benefit from PSA screening at an earlier age and at shorter intervals compared with the general male population."

Race

The United States incidence and mortality data for prostate cancer also reflect racial differences. In particular, African Americans, who are more likely to develop and die from all types of cancer than persons of any other racial and ethnic group, seem to have a significant increase in prostate cancer risk. The incidence of prostate cancer in the African American population is 275 per 100,000. This is significantly higher than the next highest risk racial group, whites, which has a prostate cancer incidence of 173 per 100,000. Mortality is also higher in African Americans, with 75 per 100,000 dying as compared to 33 per 100,000 of whites (American Cancer Society, 2003). It is unclear whether or not this variation is based on genetic or environmental factors; however, African American men have a higher incidence of prostate cancer than do black men in Africa or Asia (Pienta and Esper, 1993). While the greater incidence of cancer in general among African Americans has been shown to be affected by their disproportionate distribution at lower socioeconomic levels, in the case of prostate cancer lower socioeconomic status has not been shown to significantly increase the risk of prostate cancer in African Americans (Baquet et al., 1991; Pienta and Esper, 1993).

Diet

A high-fat diet has long been suspected to be a risk factor in prostate cancer. Evidence suggests that some aspect of dietary fat intake contributes to the variation in prostate cancer rates worldwide and to the changes in risk following migration (Gann et al., 1994). Fat may increase the risk of prostate cancer through several mechanisms. First, fat can alter androgen levels. Men who consumed less fat had lower plasma testosterone levels in a number of studies. Second, fat may be a source of free radicals. Third, proinflammatory fatty acid metabolites may be carcinogenic. Several studies have shown a correlation between increased dietary fat and increased prostate cancer risk but it has not been proven definitively (Reiter and dekernion, 2002).

Cigarette Smoking

There is little agreement over the role of cigarette smoking in prostate cancer risk (Reiter and deKernion, 2002). Cigarette smoking, while a common risk factor for lung and bladder cancer, has been shown in some studies to add little, if anything to the risk of developing prostate cancer (Pienta and Esper, 1993). As gay men smoke at far higher rates than the general population of men, 42% as compared to 29%, this may affect their risk of prostate cancer but no studies have shown this definitively (Dean et al., 2000).

Infectious Agents

Infectious agents have also been discussed in the literature in terms of their potential to increase the risk of prostate cancer. As Reiter and deKernion (2002) write, "Sexual activity, for example, is hypothesized to expose the prostate to infectious agents, which may increase the risk of prostate cancer, akin to the causal relationship between human papillomavirus (HPV) and cervical cancer in women. Although some studies have found a link among early sexual intercourse, number of sexual partners, and prostate cancer, these results have not been consistent. Studies have also not consistently identified HPV or other pathogens (i.e., chlamydia) in prostate cancer tissue."

SCREENING

Prostate cancer screening is one of the most contentious medical issues in both the professional and lay media. Seldom does a week go by without some study either advocating for or against prostate-specific antigen (PSA) testing. For example, the Centers for Disease Control and Prevention (CDC) posits the following: The "CDC does not recommend routine screening for prostate cancer because there is no scientific consensus on whether screening and treatment of early stage prostate cancer reduces mortality" (Center for Disease Control and Prevention, 2003). The American Cancer Society, on the other hand, recommends a PSA test and a digital rectal examination (DRE) annually beginning at age fifty for men with a life expectancy of at least ten years. Their guidelines also call for men at high risk, which they define as African Americans or men who have a first-degree relative diagnosed with prostate cancer at a young age, to begin PSA testing and DREs at age 45 (American Cancer Society, 2003). In the absence of a definitive, universal recommendation, each man must make the decision in consultation with his doctor. However, "most authors agree that it is plausible that aggressive screening and treatment are responsible for the decreases in prostate cancer mortality" (Reiter and deKernion, 2002). Currently the American Urological Association guidelines recommend a yearly PSA test and DRE starting at age 50 and for men at high-risk at age 40; this seems to make the most sense right now.

Once the decision has been made to undergo a PSA test and a DRE, the doctor and patient must potentially wade into the next debate: at what PSA level is a biopsy of the prostate advisable? If the patient has an abnormal DRE, the answer is clear: a biopsy should be performed (Terris, 2002). However, the debate occurs when the DRE is normal and the PSA is elevated. A PSA threshold of 4 ng/mL has usually been used; however, the PSA threshold that balances the goals of reducing prostate cancer mortality and reducing unnecessary biopsies is not known. In fact, 25% of men with cancer have PSA levels less than 4 ng/mL (Carter and Partin, 2002). Using a threshold level below 4 ng/mL may detect prostate cancer more frequently in its curable stages, but will also mean more biopsies and may detect more harmless cancers (Catalona et al., 2000). In addition, normal PSA levels increase as men age, so doctors need to take into account patient age, along with other risk factors, as noted above, when evaluating the proper threshold PSA level at which a biopsy is recommended. The screening studies done by Catalona and his associates (Catalona et al., 2000) specifically suggest that, "a 2.6 ng/mL PSA cutoff detects more potentially curable cancers without over detecting harmless ones." However, the authors go on to say that definitions of curable cancers vary; their study included only men with organ-confined disease and clear surgical margins. A review of 36,316 prostate biopsies from 1997 through 2002 indicates that the risk of detecting prostate cancer is 27.5% in men with PSA levels of 2.5 to 4.0 ng/mL and 30.1% for men with PSA levels of 4.0 to 10.0 ng/mL (Lowe, 2003). Therefore, our recommendation is that any man under age 60 with a PSA level of greater than 2.5 ng/mL should have a prostate biopsy.

The prostate biopsy is the gold standard for prostate cancer diagnosis. As patients commonly undergo a biopsy with both a normal DRE finding and ultrasound images, the doctor is not targeting a specific potential tumor. Instead, doctors take 6 to 14 samples from various areas of the prostate, which allows them to gather information on the prostate as a whole (Terris, 2002). The samples are evaluated and any observed cancers are classified using the Gleason scale. The Gleason system is based on the glandular pattern of the tumor and each sample is given a score from 1 to 5 (1 being the most differentiated and 5 being the least differentiated). Differentiation refers to whether or not the cells have distinct, clearly defined borders under microscopic evaluation. Well-differentiated cancers (a low Gleason level) tend to progress very slowly, while "poorly differentiated cancers tend to spread like wildfire" (Walsh and Worthington, 2001). The scores of the two primary patterns revealed are added together to give the patient a Gleason score of somewhere from 2 to 10 (Epstein, 2002). As described above, the Gleason score establishes the aggressivity of the tumor, with a score of

2-6 generally implying a good prognosis, 7 being uncertain and scores of 8 through 10 indicating aggressive and dangerous cancers.

Once the Gleason score is calculated and a definitive diagnosis of prostate cancer is established, the doctor will evaluate the data along with an estimation of the stage of a cancer. The stage depends on whether the cancer can be felt during the DRE and, if so, the expected extent of the cancer: Nonpalpable tumor [T1], palpable tumor confined to the prostate [T2], or palpable tumor beyond the prostate [T3]. Armed with the patient's Gleason score, his PSA level, and the clinical stage, the physician can now use the Partin tables to arrive at a pre-treatment estimate for the patient's probable disease spread. The Partin tables give probabilities of a final pathologic stage, which includes information about whether or not the cancer is organ-confined or has penetrated the capsule, in addition to the status of the seminal vesicles and the lymph nodes. This information is then used to counsel the patient with respect to treatment alternatives and probability of complete eradication of the tumor (Carter and Partin, 2002).

TREATMENTS

Following a diagnosis of prostate cancer, the patient and his doctor must make a decision as to the optimal course of treatment. Treatments can be broken down into three categories. First, therapies with a curative intent. These include radical prostatectomy, radiation, which includes both external beam and brachytherapy [implanted radioactive seeds], cryotherapy or a combination of the above. The second class of therapies is hormonal. Hormonal therapy is aimed at achieving testosterone inhibition via surgical or medical castration. Hormone therapy seeks to take advantage of the fact that most prostate cancers are, at least initially, endocrine-dependent tumors (Schröder, 2002). The third therapy is watchful waiting, which, as the name implies, involves monitoring the patient for disease progression while undertaking no treatment with the hope that the disease progression in that particular patient will be slow enough so as not to affect his life expectancy.

Radical Prostatectomy

During a radical prostatectomy, the entire prostate gland and seminal vesicles are removed. For men with prostate cancer contained within the prostate, in good general health and having a life expectancy of greater than ten years, it is the gold standard of treatments. A nationwide survey indicated that 95% of American urologists would recommend radical prostatectomy for patients aged 70 years or less with localized disease (Eastham and Scardino, 2002; Kirby, 1998).

The surgery can be performed either retropubically (through the abdomen), perineally (through the area between the scrotum and the anus) or, more recently, laparoscopically (using a lighted tube that enters the body through a tiny hole, through which a surgeon can thread a scalpel).

Several factors speak in favor of a radical prostatectomy once a patient is deemed a candidate for the procedure. First, it can definitively remove the cancer if it is contained within the prostate. Second, the removal and full analysis of the prostate allows for a thorough evaluation of the cancer, which can allow for better prognosis determination. Third, due to surgical advances in the last twenty years, the surgery is usually able to preserve the nerve bundles controlling erectile function if the cancer has not spread to them (Eastham and Scardino, 2002).

Disadvantages of a radical prostatectomy are that it is major inpatient surgery that can involve bleeding and complications with general anesthesia, incontinence, and potential persistent erectile dysfunction. All of these risks can be greatly minimized by having the surgery performed by a competent urological surgeon (Eastham and Scardino, 2002).

In terms of incontinence, fewer than 10% of patients that have the surgery done by someone with experience have significant incontinence after surgery. At 2 years post-operatively, one study showed that only 5% of patients were not dry. Factors such as younger age, preservation of both nerve bundles and surgical technique are the greatest prognostic factors for incontinence (Eastham and Scardino, 2002).

Erectile dysfunction is also a risk with a radical prostatectomy. Recovery of erectile function is directly correlated with patient age, preoperative potency and the extent of nerve bundle preservation. For a man younger than sixty with preoperative erections and with a bilateral nerve sparing operation, there is a 76% chance of recovery of potency by three years post-op. Those rates decline with increasing age, nerve bundle damage or removal, and other potency affecting diseases (such as diabetes and hypertension) (Eastham and Scardino, 2002).

In addition to potential complications, the doctor and patient must determine the chance that the patient has of being cured by the surgery. The status of the patient post-op is generally measured through periodic PSA testing. With the removal of the prostate, the expectation and hope is that the patient's PSA will remain at undetectable levels. When the PSA climbs, it is referred to as biochemical recurrence and means that some of the cancer remained in the patient after surgery. Approximately 35% of men will experience a detectable PSA rise within ten years following surgery (Pound et al., 1999; Roberts et al., 2001). Factors that affect the chances of recurrence are patient age, post-op surgical margins (whether the cancer appeared contained within the prostate gland), Gleason score and pre-op PSA. A recent study comparing patient age and recurrence rates showed that patients younger than 70 had almost half the risk of recurrence as those over 70 (Öbek et al., 1999). In terms of the impact of the Gleason score on recurrence, one study showed rates of recurrence from 20% for patients with Gleason scores of two to five up to 78% for Gleason scores of eight through ten (Roberts et al., 2001).

Radiation Therapy

Radiation therapy is also used in the treatment of early stage prostate cancer. Patients who are candidates for radiotherapy tend to be patients with localized cancer with a life expectancy of seven to ten years or more for whom surgery is either not suitable or not desired. The two main radiotherapy techniques are external radiation therapy (XRT) and brachytherapy (seed implant therapy). Both therapies are radical in nature and seek to destroy the prostate and prostate cancer cells. However, the prostate is not actually removed and so recurrence rates tend to be higher (3% to 40%) with radiation therapy than radical prostatectomy (Kirby, 1998).

XRT involves electron beam radiation treatments that are generally given for five days per week over a six to eight week period. The actual dose takes only minutes to deliver. Seeding involves the surgical implantation of small radioactive pellets into the prostate gland, under regional (spinal) or general anesthesia.

The primary advantage of radiotherapy is that the patient avoids major surgery and the complications therein. XRT treatments are painless, quick, and can be performed in an outpatient center. Likewise, the implantation of the seeds takes only one or two hours and usually involves a hospital stay of less than one day. The pain and discomfort from the seeding is generally minor and lasts for only a few days; however, dysuria (pain during urination) and urgency can last for several months.

The disadvantages of radiotherapy, apart from the many hospital visits required for XRT, are risks of urinary frequency and burning, chronic bowel complications, incontinence, and sexual side effects. In addition, seeding can lead to rectal bleeding in a small proportion of patients, fewer than 5%. Erectile dysfunction after radical prostatectomy is usually immediate and tends to improve over months and years; patients who undergo radiotherapy may find that their sexual function decreases over time. One study at the University of Chicago showed that 53% of previously potent men in the study reported impotence by sixty months post external beam radiation treatments (D'Amico et al., 2002). Another study directly comparing sexual function and sexual bother (the degree of interference or annoyance caused by any limitations in sexual function) in pelvic irradiation versus radical prostatectomy came up with similar conclusions. The authors found that while sexual function was higher in radiotherapy patients one year post-treatment, by the end of the second year radical prostatectomy patients reported higher sexual function scores as compared to the radiotherapy population studied. As the authors wrote, "Both our study and theirs confirm the common clinical observation that long-term sexual function outcomes are similar in this population, regardless of whether RP or XRT (pelvic irradiation) is selected as primary therapy" (Litwin et al., 1999).

In comparing XRT with seeding, a 2000 editorial in the journal *Urology* (Hanks, 2000) strongly advocated for XRT over seeding. Hanks writes, "we must rely on the available evidence demonstrating the superiority of external beam radiation therapy over implants for patients with prostate cancer and a favorable prognosis. This advantage is particularly evident in a major reduction of late urinary tract morbidity, with 2% of patients wearing pads versus 16% after implants and no urinary diversions versus 2.5% to 3.5% after implants."

Cryotherapy

Cryotherapy involves the insertion of probes containing liquid argon gas into the prostate. The gland is then frozen and thawed causing cellular necrosis and sloughing of the prostate cancer and gland. While less invasive than a radical prostatectomy, high rates of complications have prevented widespread adoption of cryotherapy as a treatment. Complications include rectal freezing or fistula, urethral sloughing, urinary incontinence, and impotence (Kirby, 1998). Impotence rates of 80% or higher have been reported due to the extension of the ice ball formed by the procedure, which goes beyond the prostate gland, into the area of the neurovascular bundles. In addition, one study shows that impotence after the procedure is due to both nerve and blood vessel injury. Post-cryosurgery, impotence should be expected. Incontinence rates have been shown to be as high as 70%, especially after prior radiation therapy (Shinohara and Carroll, 2002).

Hormonal Therapy

Hormonal therapy is palliative rather than curative and has become the primary therapy of choice in advanced disease and in cancer that has spread to the lymph nodes or bone. For localized prostate cancer, hormonal therapy has traditionally only been considered for older men who do not want or are unable to undergo radical therapy. Hormonal therapy is also being investigated in combination with surgery or radiation (Kirby, 1998).

Hormone therapy relies on the fact that male hormones, particularly testosterone, influence prostate cancer initiation and progression. Prostate tumors are "exquisitely sensitive to androgens and regress after medical or surgical castration" (Reiter and deKernion, 2002). By using drugs to block the hormone production (medical castration) or through surgical castration, symptoms are eliminated in the most symptomatic patients; clinical progression is delayed and there is the possibility of prolonging life. Eventually, however, those prostate cancer cells that do not depend on androgens tend to multiply and threaten the patient's life.

Medical castration is generally preferred by patients, both for the reduced psychological impact as well as the reversibility of the treatment. Disadvantages of hormone therapy include hot flashes, decreased libido, erectile dysfunction, osteoporosis, reduced muscle mass, anemia, and decreased mental acuity. Impotence, however, is not a certainty. According to Walsh and Worthington (2001), ten percent of men remain potent (in this case impotence meaning loss of libido as well as erectile function).

Diet and Alternative Therapies

As discussed above, there is evidence linking the development of prostate cancer to dietary factors. Partly due to this, many patients turn to changes in diet as a way to prevent or treat their prostate cancer. In particular, patients frequently take selenium (200 mcg/day) and vitamin E (400 IU/day) for prevention of the disease. Neither of these supplements is seen as a treatment for confirmed prostate cancer but they are frequently taken as an adjunct after one of the definitive therapies above. In the same vein, many patients increase their intake of soy products (e.g., tofu, soy milk) and lycopene (tomatoes) in order to take advantage of the potential health benefits of both nutrients. In the absence of definitive proof of their effectiveness, supplementing a definitive therapy with diet changes may make sense.

Some patients focus on a mind-body connection in order to affect the course of their disease. While patients must avoid the inclination to punish themselves if the disease progresses negatively, many patients will find that a positive outlook and attitude can have a significant impact on their emotional well being during treatment.

GAY MEN AND PROSTATE CANCER

As mentioned above, gay men, beyond having a significant chance of having to deal with prostate cancer in either themselves or their partner, have several specific issues that need to be dealt with by health providers in order to ensure proper care.

Anabolic Steroids

The use of anabolic steroids in the gay male population is probably higher than the general male population due to several factors. First, steroids are being prescribed to gay men with AIDS as part of their treatment. The drugs replenish testosterone levels and help to fight fatigue, weight loss, and low sex drive. Second, Yeland and Tiggemann (2003) suggest that the gay 'ideal' often involves being thin and muscular, a fact that encourages some gay men to use steroids as a performance enhancer. In two separate surveys of gay gym patrons in London, 13.5% and 15.2% of the men questioned, respectively, reported that they were current users of anabolic steroids (Bolding et al., 1999; 2002).

When steroid use is combined with prostate cancer, the results can be devastating. Many men may have latent prostate cancers that are insignificant and will never affect their lives. Walsh and Worthington (2001) state that in such cases using steroids "could be like pouring kerosene on a fire. It should go without saying that any man who has had prostate cancer should *never* take any form of male hormone supplementation." They go on to recommend that any man at risk of developing prostate cancer have a needle biopsy prior to any medical treatment of low testosterone (Jackson, 2005).

Propecia (Finasteride)

Finasteride is marketed as Proscar (5 mg), a treatment for an enlarged prostate gland. In a lower dosage it is available as Propecia (1 mg), a hair-loss treatment. While there is no data suggesting that gay men are greater users of Propecia than straight men, Merck, the manufacturer of the drug, has been directly targeting the gay community as a potential market for the drug since 2000 (Goetzl, 2000).

A problem with the drug as it relates to prostate cancer is that it lowers a patient's PSA. If a doctor is screening for prostate cancer using a PSA test and is unaware of the patient's use of finasteride, prostate cancer will be under-diagnosed. The prescribing information for the drug states, "until further information is gathered in men > 41 years of age without benign prostatic hyperplasia (BPH), consideration should be given to doubling the PSA level in men undergoing this test while taking Propecia" (Merck, 1997). This recommendation is given scientific support by Andriole et al. (1998) who suggest that when the use of finasteride is ascertained "multiplying PSA by 2 and using normal ranges for untreated men preserves the usefulness of PSA for prostate cancer detection."

The role of finasteride in prostate cancer was the focus of a recent study that concluded that finasteride in 5 mg doses might actually prevent or delay the appearance of prostate cancer. However, these benefits must be weighed against sexual side effects and an increased risk of high-grade prostate cancer (Thompson et al., 2003).

HIV/AIDS

In states that report HIV infection, men who have sex with men represent 38% of all newly reported cases (Dean et al., 2000). Thus any doctor treating a gay patient for prostate cancer needs to be aware of several issues in regards to HIV and prostate cancer.

Several cancers are included as AIDS-defining diseases. Prostate cancer has never been included in that group. While there has been no definitive evidence, there is some reason to believe that the risk of prostate cancer is higher in patients with HIV infection (Cooksley et al., 1999; Crum et al., 2002; Santos et al., 2002). While it may not necessarily increase prostate cancer, HIV may increase the possibility that the immune system will not be able to fight the disease. The fact that the immune system may play a role in prostate cancer has encouraged researchers to look at using immunotherapy as a way to enhance conventional prostate cancer treatments (Kaminski et al., 2003). In addition to potentially increasing the risk of prostate cancer, the disease also appears to be more virulent in HIV infected patients; this was true in those who were already hypogonadal (low testosterone level) from their HIV disease at the time of their prostate cancer diagnosis (Kwan and Lowe, 1995). This population would probably be served well by increased screening beginning at earlier ages such as is recommended for those in other high risk groups.

One factor in deciding whether or not to treat prostate cancer and which treatment to choose is the life expectancy of the patient. With the dramatically reduced life expectancies of AIDS patients in the early stages of the epidemic, doctors tended to offer radiation as a treatment choice instead of radical prostatectomy, the latter being generally not advised if the patient's life expectancy was less than ten years. The primary treatment options had traditionally been radiation or seeding instead of hormonal because HIV patients did not respond well to hormonal treatments (Kwan and Lowe, 1995). As the use of highly active antiretroviral therapy (HAART) became widespread in 1996, the life expectancy of patients increased and thus doctors now include the option of a radical prostatectomy when helping a patient decide on their prostate cancer treatment (Levinson, Nagler, and Lowe, 2005).

PSA Test/Anal Intercourse

Any PSA test is only as good as the conditions under which the sample was taken. Several studies have shown that certain urologic procedures can increase the PSA level in a patient and these elevated readings may affect a patient's medical decisions. While many sources cite that the PSA test should be taken from a patient prior to a digital rectal examination, there is reason to believe that the DRE does not have that significant an impact on PSA (Klein and Lowe, 1997). However, a vigorous prostate massage, "may affect the serum PSA significantly; therefore it is prudent to measure the serum PSA before prostate massage or to wait at least three days for the PSA to return to baseline" (Klein and Lowe, 1997). This finding would seem to bear on how the patient's engaging in receptive anal intercourse might affect their PSA test. Ejaculation will also affect PSA levels. Thus, knowing the affect of prostatic massage and ejaculation on PSA levels, it would be prudent to assume that a patient should probably refrain from receptive anal intercourse and ejaculation for at least forty-eight hours prior to a PSA test.

Doctor-Patient Communication

Prostate cancer does more to a man than threaten his life. Because of its location near the reproductive and urinary systems and the impact of treatments, it has the potential to affect his sexuality, sense of masculinity and self-esteem. All of these are significant psychological issues that can affect a patient's recovery. Gay patients face the added burden of revealing their sexual practices and dealing with potential homophobia in the medical setting. The burden usually falls on the patient to tell the doctor that he is gay. This is not helped by the fact that intake forms covering sexual history rarely include the option for providing information on same-sex partners. One study on lesbian and gay health found, "disclosure of sexual orientation in a health care setting remains infrequent for the majority of gay men and lesbians" (Dean et al., 2000).

If a gay patient is partnered but does not feel comfortable being out to his healthcare provider, he is likely to experience incremental psychic anguish and a loss of benefits that might accrue from including his partner in treatment decisions and recovery. As studies with heterosexual couples have shown, the spouse of a cancer patient experiences at least as much psychological distress as the patient (Heyman and Rosner, 1996). In the case of a closeted gay patient who does not feel comfortable including his partner, the stresses are exacerbated for both parties.

Prostate cancer requires an active participation of the patient and his support network. From the initial diagnosis, the patient is traditionally provided with a selection of treatment options and a man may feel "both an urgency to act and an inability to act" (Heyman and Rosner, 1996). Studies have shown that female partners in this situation provide an invaluable support system. While they seem to leave the final decision up to the patient, wives take on roles of gathering information, taking notes in meeting, and asking questions. As Heyman and Rosner (1996) wrote, "She [the wife] became the conduit for information between the professionals and her husband." Their study also concludes that, "couples view the wife as a partner in managing the disease and expect that she may even act on behalf of her husband. When this role is not legitimized by the physician, the relationship with that physician may be jeopardized." It is not a difficult leap to imagine what the affect of the loss of a partner's active support could mean for a gay man in this situation.

Another study by Srirangam et al. (2003) specifically attempted to understand the influence of the partner on the treatment choice in early prostate cancer. While the study also found that partners deliberately left the final treatment decision to the patient, 93% of the patients in the study reported consulting their partners before making their final treatment decision and 88% of the partners felt that they were actively involved in the decision-making process. The value of the partner's input is obviously affected by their involvement in the process. It is the partner's invitation to add his interpretation of the information gathered that helps the patient formulate a final decision; but if the partner is excluded, because of homophobic reasons emanating from the doctor and/ or the patient, his input is less likely to be valued. Srirangam et al. (2003) also found that 48% of the partners felt the experience of dealing with the patient's prostate cancer had brought them closer, 34% felt there had been no change, and the remaining 18% admitted feelings of helplessness and strain. The authors add that, "We therefore strongly recommend that the onus is put on the medical staff to include both patient and partner when informing the former of the diagnosis, and at subsequent clinic visits during the decision-making process." In the case of gay men this may be difficult as the lack of desire to disclose sexuality and sexual orientation is influenced, not merely by the provider, but also by the patient who may have very strong feelings about revealing his sexual behaviors and orientation to his doctor.

In terms of sexual side effects of treatments, many studies have been conducted regarding post-treatment erectile dysfunction, its amelioration and its psychological consequences. However, gay men who engage in receptive anal intercourse may also face the sometimes-painful reality of diminished sexual stimulation due to the removal of the prostate. Doctors may not generally discuss this topic, but when counseling a gay man as to how his post-treatment sexuality will be affected, an omission of this fact can cause some patient post-treatment distress (Goldstone, 2005).

It has been shown that patient attitude has a real impact on the patient's perception of what is bothersome about treatment side effects. If because of lack of disclosure the patient is missing partner involvement and thus inadvertently increasing the stress on his personal relationship, it would be expected that he might also face increased distress from any subsequent treatment side-effects. This seems to be an unwise and unnecessary burden for a patient and his partner to bear.

CONCLUSION

Prostate cancer will be a fact of life for a large segment of the male population. While cancer does not discriminate between gay men, straight men, partnered men or single men, those men in partnerships face a high likelihood of dealing with the direct effect of prostate cancer on their own or their partner's health and sexuality. That being said, the medical community and patients themselves need to ensure open communication so that issues specifically affecting them as gay men are addressed and so that unnecessary stress is avoided in what will undoubtedly be one of the most stressful times in a man's life. Finally, gay men should be treated with the same respect and concern as the general population regarding prostate cancer screening, evaluation and treatment regardless of their sexual orientation or HIV status.

REFERENCES

American Cancer Society (2004), *Cancer Facts & Figures 2004*.

Andriole, G., Guess, H., Epstein, J., Wise, H., Kadmon, D., Crawford, E., Hudson, P., Jackson, C., Romas, N., Patterson, L., Cook, T. & Waldstreicher, J. (1998), Treatment with finasteride preserves usefulness of prostate-specific antigen in the detection of prostate cancer: results of a randomized, double-blind, placebo-controlled clinical trial. *Urology*, 52:195-202.

Baquet, C., Horm, J., Gibbs, T. & Greenwald, P. (1991), Socioeconomic factors and cancer incidence among blacks and whites. *J. Natl. Cancer Inst.*, 83: 551-557.

Bolding, G., Sherr, L., Maguire, M. & Elford, J. (1999), HIV risk behaviours among gay men who use anabolic steroids. *Addiction*, 94:1829-1835.

Bolding, G., Sherr, L. & Elford, J. (2002), Use of anabolic steroids and associated health risks among gay men attending London gyms. *Addiction*, 97:195-203.

Carter, H. & Partin, A. (2002), Diagnosis and staging of prostate cancer. In: *Campbell's Urology. 8th ed.*, eds: P. Walsh, A. Retik & E. Vaughn. Philadelphia, PA: WB Saunders, pp. 3055-3079.

Catalona, W., Ramos, C., Carvalhal, G. & Yan, Y. (2000), Lowering PSA cutoffs to enhance detection of curable prostate cancer. *Urology*, 55:791-795.

Centers for Disease Control and Prevention (2003), Prostate Cancer: The Public Health Perspective. Washington, DC: Author.

Cooksley, C., Hwang, L., Waller, D. & Ford, C. (1999), HIV-related malignancies: Community-based study using linkage of cancer registry and HIV registry data. *International J. STD & AIDS*, 10:795-802.

Crum, N., Hale, B., Utz, G. & Wallace, M. (2002), Increased risk of prostate cancer in HIV infection? *AIDS*, 16:1703-1704.

D'Amico, A., Crook, J., Beard, C., DeWeese, T., Hurwitz, M. & Kaplan, I. (2002), Radiation therapy for prostate cancer. In: *Campbell's Urology. 8th ed.*, eds: P. Walsh, A. Retik & E. Vaughn. Philadelphia, PA: WB Saunders, pp. 3147-3170.

Dean, L., Meyer, I., Robinson, K., Sell, R., Sember, R., Silenzio, V., Bowen, D., Bradford, J., Rothblum, E., Scout, White, J., Dunn, P., Lawrence, A., Wolfe, D. & Xavier, J. (2000), Lesbian, gay, bisexual, and transgender health: Findings and Concerns. *J. Gay & Lesbian Medical Association*, 4:101-151.

Eastham, J. & Scardino, P. (2002), Radical Prostatectomy. In: *Campbell's Urology. 8th ed.*, eds: P. Walsh, A. Retik & E. Vaughn. Philadelphia, PA: WB Saunders, pp. 3080-3106.

Epstein, J. (2002), Pathology of prostatic neoplasia. In: *Campbell's Urology. 8th ed.*, eds: P. Walsh, A. Retik & E. Vaughn. Philadelphia, PA: WB Saunders, 86:3025-3037.

Gann, P., Hennekens, C., Sacks, F., Grodstein, F., Giovannucci, E. & Stempfer, M. (1994), Prospective study of plasma fatty acids and risk of prostate cancer. *J. Natl. Cancer Inst.*, 86:281-286.

Goetzl, D. (2000), Propecia aims $2 mil push at gay men. *Advertising Age*, 71(12):8.

Goldstone, S. E. (2005), The ups and downs of gay sex after prostate cancer treatment. *J. Gay & Lesbian Psychotherapy*, 9(1/2):43-55.

Hanks, G. (2000), The case for external beam treatment of early-stage prostate cancer. *Urology*, 55:301-305.

Heyman, E. & Rosner, T. (1996), Prostate cancer: An intimate view from patients and wives. *Urol. Nurs.*, 16:37-44.

Jackson, L. (2005), Surviving yet another challenge. *J. Gay & Lesbian Psychotherapy*, 9(1/2): 101-107.

Jemal, A., Thomas, A., Murray, T. & Thun, M. (2002), Cancer statistics, 2002. *CA Cancer J. Clin.*, 52:23-47.

Kaminski, J., Summers, J., Ward, M., Huber, M. & Minev, B. (2003), Immunotherapy and prostate cancer. *Cancer Treatment Reviews*, 29:199-209.

Kirby, R. (1998), Treatment options for early prostate cancer. *Urology*, 52:948-962.

Klein, L. & Lowe, F. (1997), The effects of prostatic manipulation on prostate-specific antigen levels. *Urol. Clin. N. America*, 24:293-297.

Kwan, D. & Lowe, F. (1995), Genitourinary manifestations of the acquired immunodeficiency syndrome. *Urology*, 45:13-27.

Levinson, A., Nagler, E. & Lowe, F. (2005), The approach to management of localized prostate cancer in patients with Immunodeficiency Syndrome. *Urology*, 65, in press.

Litwin, M., Flanders, S., Pasta, D., Stoddard, M., Lubeck, D. & Henning, J. (1999), Sexual function and bother after radical prostatectomy or radiation for prostate cancer: Multivariate quality-of-life analysis from CaPSURE. *Urology*, 54:503-508.

Lowe, F., Cavallo, C. & Kahane, H. (2003), Epidemiological evidence suggesting a PSA cut-point of 2.5 ng/mL for initiating a prostate biopsy: A review of 36,316 patients with biopsy and PSA data. *J. Urol.*, 169:Abstract DP 12,341.

Merck & Co., Inc. (1997), Propecia (Finasteride) full prescribing information. Whitehouse Station, NJ.

Öbek, C., Lai, S., Sadek, S., Civantos, F. & Soloway, M. (1999), Age as a prognostic factor for disease recurrence after radical prostatectomy. *Urology*, 54:533-538.

Pienta, K. & Esper, P. (1993), Risk factors for prostate cancer. *Ann. Intern. Med.*, 118:793-803.

Pound, C., Partin, A., Eisenberger, M., Chan, D., Pearson, J. & Walsh, P. (1999), Natural history of progression after PSA elevation following radical prostatectomy. *JAMA*, 281:1591-1597.

Reiter, R. & deKernion, J. (2002), Epidemiology, etiology, and prevention of prostate cancer. In: *Campbell's Urology. 8th ed.*, eds: P. Walsh, A. Retik & E. Vaughn. Philadelphia, PA: WB Saunders, 85:3003-3024.

Roberts, S., Blute, M., Bergstralh, E., Slezak, J. & Zincke, H. (2001), PSA doubling time as a predictor of clinical progression after biochemical failure following radical prostatectomy for prostate cancer. *Mayo Clin. Proc.*, 76:576-581.

Santos, J., Palacios, R., Ruiz, J., González, M. & Márquez, M. (2002), Unusual malignant tumours in patients with HIV infection. *International J. STD & AIDS*, 13: 674-676.

Schröder, F. (2002), Hormonal therapy of prostate cancer. In: *Campbell's Urology. 8th ed.*, eds: P. Walsh, A. Retik & E. Vaughn. Philadelphia, PA: WB Saunders, 94:3182-3208.

Shinohara, K. & Carroll, P. (2002), Cryotherapy for prostate cancer. In: *Campbell's Urology. 8th ed.*, eds: P. Walsh, A. Retik & E. Vaughn. Philadelphia, PA: WB Saunders, pp. 3171-3181.

Srirangam, S., Pearson, E., Grose, C., Brown, S., Collins, G. & O'Reilly, P. (2003), Partner's influence on patient preference for treatment in early prostate cancer. *BJU Int.*, 92:365-369.

Steinberg, G., Carter, B., Beaty, T., Childs, B. & Walsh, P. (1990), Family history and the risk of prostate cancer. *The Prostate*, 17:337-347.

Terris, M. (2002), Ultrasonography and biopsy of the prostate. In: *Campbell's Urology. 8th ed.*, eds: P. Walsh, A. Retik & E. Vaughn. Philadelphia, PA: WB Saunders, pp. 3038-3054.

Thompson, I., Goodman, P., Tangen, C., Lucia, M., Miller, G., Ford, L., Lieber, M., Cespedes, R., Atkins, J., Lippman, S., Carlin, S., Ryan, A., Szczepanek, C., Crowley, J. & Coltman, C. (2003), The influence of finasteride on the development of prostate cancer. *N. Engl. J. Med.*, 349:215-24.

Walsh, P. & Worthington, J. (2001), *Dr. Patrick Walsh's Guide to Surviving Prostate Cancer*. New York, NY: Warner Books.

Yeland, C. & Tiggemann, M. (2003), Muscularity and the gay ideal: Body dissatisfaction and disordered eating in homosexual men. *Eating Behaviors*, 4:107-116.

Zeegers, M., Jellema, A. & Ostrer, H. (2003), Empiric risk of prostate carcinoma for relatives of patients with prostate carcinoma. *Cancer*, 97:1894-1903.

A Gay Urologist's Changing Views
on Prostate Cancer

David Cornell, MD

SUMMARY. As the voluminous data linking PSA and pathology results have accumulated, more refined diagnostic algorithms have resulted. These paradigms may lead to diagnosis of extremely low volume prostate cancers. The author offers his own conclusions in regard to diagnostic tests, treatment options, and managing lifestyle-impacting side effects of treatment. He offers observations from his own practice as an openly gay urologist about the ways in which prostate cancer affects gay men and his development of an Internet group for gay men with prostate cancer. The importance of active involvement in one's diagnosis and treatment is also stressed. *[Article copies available for a fee from The Haworth Document Delivery Service: 1-800-HAWORTH. E-mail address: <docdelivery@haworthpress.com> Website: <http://www.HaworthPress.com> © 2005 by The Haworth Press, Inc. All rights reserved.]*

KEYWORDS. AIDS, benign prostatic hypertrophy (BPH), gay, Gleason score, HIV, homosexuality, impotence, incontinence, Internet, support group, Partin tables, prostate cancer, PSA, PSA velocity, radical prostatectomy (RP), urologist

---

David Cornell is a Diplomate of the American Board of Urology and is in private practice in Atlanta, GA.

[Haworth co-indexing entry note]: "A Gay Urologist's Changing Views on Prostate Cancer." Cornell, David. Co-published simultaneously in *Journal of Gay & Lesbian Psychotherapy* (The Haworth Medical Press, an imprint of The Haworth Press, Inc.) Vol. 9, No. 1/2, 2005, pp. 29-41; and: *A Gay Man's Guide to Prostate Cancer* (ed: Gerald Perlman, and Jack Drescher) The Haworth Medical Press, an imprint of The Haworth Press, Inc., 2005, pp. 29-41. Single or multiple copies of this article are available for a fee from The Haworth Document Delivery Service [1-800-HAWORTH, 9:00 a.m. - 5:00 p.m. (EST). E-mail address: docdelivery@haworthpress.com].

http://www.haworthpress.com/web/JGLP
© 2005 by The Haworth Press, Inc. All rights reserved.
Digital Object Identifier: 10.1300/J236v09n01_03

HISTORICAL PERSPECTIVE

The diagnosis and management of prostate cancer has long been and still remains one of the more controversial topics in urology. There is no consensus of opinion about the ideal mode of treatment and thoughts about treatment are under constant reevaluation. Consideration of a strategy for the diagnosis and treatment of prostate cancer should acknowledge this controversy and reflect upon the history of medicine and urology as it relates to this disease.

Prostate cancer was a largely neglected disease until the mid 1980s. There was no method for early detection, as PSA testing was not available. Diagnosis was only suspected by digital rectal exam (DRE) and confirmed by finger directed biopsy using archaic and not very patient-friendly instruments. About one-third of the newly-diagnosed cases came to the physician's attention because of symptomatic metastatic disease. This most frequently represented spread into the bones of the lower back (lumbosacral vertebrae) which caused severe lower back pain. Nearly half of patients presented with prostate cancer that had already escaped cure (Whitmore, 1984).

Many others without frank metastatic disease had cancer that had advanced beyond curability. Nor did the men who might have been candidates for treatment have available any of today's advanced techniques, i.e., nerve-sparing radical prostatectomy, ultrasound-directed brachytherapy (radiation seed implants), or cryotherapy. Radical prostatectomy was technically crude, often resulting in blood transfusions, and frequently leaving the patient incontinent of urine and sexually impotent. Seeding of the prostate was done through an abdominal incision and was guided by the radiotherapist's finger rather than ultrasound. Consequently, rectal complications were not rare and seed distribution was extremely irregular. External beam radiotherapy was well established and generally well tolerated but without some of its current refinement.

Thus, prostate cancer prior to the 1990s was usually detected at an advanced stage with few sophisticated treatment options available. At that time, the main argument in urology was whether or not to treat the disease at all; data suggested that treatment was not significantly altering overall survival rate (Whitmore, Warner and Thompson, 1991).

The introductions of and increasing utilization of both PSA for early detection and the refinement of the nerve-sparing radical prostatectomy technique occurred at about the same time (Walsh and Doker, 1982). During the 1990s, prostate cancer went from being relatively ignored to becoming the most prominent issue in urology. The use of PSA allowed for early diagnosis so that a much greater percentage of newly discovered patients had a probability of cure. During the decade of the 90s, the stage observed (the size and extent of tumor or tumors) at diagnosis changed dramatically. Thanks to the utilization of PSA for screening, the presence of metastatic disease at the time of diagnosis declined significantly (Schroder et al., 2000).

Physicians have learned to use PSA more effectively. At first, many clinicians utilized it to validate or refute an abnormal prostate exam. If a physician thought he palpated a nodule, he might obtain a PSA level; if the level was normal, the physician might choose to follow the patient, reserving biopsy for nodules accompanied by elevated PSA. Gradually, however, PSA came into widespread use as an annual screening test for prostate cancer. It was recommended by some physicians routinely, particularly for men in their 60s, sometimes even for men in their 50s. A prostate was assumed to be normal if the PSA level was within the lab normal range, usually less than 4.0 ng/ml. There also was a growing awareness of other conditions in the prostate associated with elevation of the PSA; the most common being prostatitis and benign prostatic hypertrophy (BHP or benign enlargement of the prostate).

With increased utilization of PSA screening during the 1990s, more data about the test was gathered and more prostate cancer diagnoses were made. The use of PSA eventually found its way into the health screening of younger men. As a result, it became understood that age adjustment of the normal test range was necessary to provide greater sensitivity for the younger group. The reason for this adjustment is that men in their 60s and 70s are expected to have a greater volume of benign prostatic hypertrophy than those in their 40s. Since benign enlargement is also reflected in higher PSA levels, a higher mean value would be expected with advancing age. Therefore the upper limit of normal for a 40-year-old is 2.0 ng/mL rather than the overall laboratory normal of 4.0 ng/mL (Oesterling et al., 1993).

As larger numbers of individuals began to accumulate PSA histories, i.e., serial values over consecutive years, another fact became apparent: A rise in the PSA value from one year to the next was suspicious for cancer. This new parameter is referred to as "PSA velocity." By following serial values in the same individual, cancers can be detected by accelerated rate of changes even before the value reaches the laboratory abnormal range. In other words, a man who has a PSA of 0.3 one year and 1.1 the following year (both apparently normal values) is nevertheless at risk for cancer and aggressive urologists will evaluate it further.

The velocity change that has been demonstrated to be statistically significant is 0.75 ng/mL/year (Carter et al., 1995).

Other diagnostic techniques and standards have also evolved over the past fifteen years. In the 1980s and early 1990s, an abnormal PSA was followed by ultrasound. Biopsies were only done of abnormal areas imaged on sonogram. By the 1990s, however, it became evident that only a small minority of prostate cancers had a sonographic abnormality. Increasing the number of biopsies increased diagnostic accuracy. In the 1990s, six biopsies were done for all men with PSA abnormalities. The current standard is 12 or more biopsies. The introduction of local anesthesia to improve patient acceptance of the ultrasound-guided biopsy technique has been another advance.

TREATMENT AND COMPLICATIONS

The results of aggressive PSA and biopsy utilization are affecting the outcome of prostate cancer treatment. When treating earlier stage smaller volume cancers it follows logically, and in practice, that outcomes improve. In the past, much data existed which demonstrated that prior to PSA early detection, medical science was not affecting the survival of prostate cancer. At that time, regardless whether the prostate cancer population was treated with radical prostatectomy, external beam radiotherapy, brachytherapy, or expectant management (watchful waiting) overall survival was not affected. The logical corollary is that a significant number of patients were being overtreated. There is a subset of prostate cancer patients who live with this cancer and have no decrease in longevity. It is not known how to identify them but that they exist is well established. This has not changed as more cases are detected. The fact that now younger, more active and productive men are being treated, is cause for some reconsideration of recommended therapy.

The result of increasing refinement in diagnosis, is that prostate cancer is being detected in younger men with lower volume disease. This creates the need to reconsider and refine treatment options since the disease is now affecting men who are still, for the most part, physically, economically, and sexually active; men who frequently present with only microscopic foci of cancer. These men–in their 40s and 50s, and sometimes even in their 30s–are not ready or willing to face sexual impotency or urinary incontinence. Many are also unwilling to consider several months' rehabilitation from major surgery. Consequently, further refinements have continued in the technique of radical prostatectomy;

and brachytherapy and cryotherapy have continued to gain popularity and credibility.

Occurring concurrently with the evolution of prostate cancer diagnosis and treatment has been refinement in the management of erectile dysfunction and urinary incontinence. This makes it possible to successfully manage the potential side effects of prostate cancer therapy. These advances include medications for impotency delivered by mouth, injection, and/or urethral suppository. There have also been improvements in penile prosthetics. For incontinence, many new medications with fewer side-effects have evolved, as well as implantable sphincter prosthetics.

A UROLOGIST'S EXPERIENCE

Having completed residency in 1985, I had experience with the archaic method of diagnosing prostate cancer by digital rectal exam. I also had considerable experience with men presenting initially with advanced metastatic cancer. Seeing men at the peak of their lives with a newly-diagnosed, incurable, fatal condition was hardly the reason I chose a career in urology. Consequently, watching metastatic disease increasingly become a rarity has been a miraculous transformation. Being able to offer cure to almost all of the prostate cancer patients who present to me is a quantum leap from the frustration of having no chance of cure for almost half of them. The emotional, financial, and physical devastation that my generation of urologists observed from the disease prior to the '90s definitely affected my thoughts and feelings about treating early stages of prostate cancer.

As the era of PSA-detected prostate cancers emerged in the late '80s and '90s, I came to believe in a very aggressive approach to treating all early disease. I steered virtually all of my patients toward radical prostatectomy. It seemed rather straightforward that radical prostatectomy was the superior therapy. If the disease was confined to the prostate, and if the prostate could be removed, why do anything else? Radiation seeding of the prostate still had a poor reputation from an earlier incarnation of the 1970s and early '80s. External beam radiotherapy was not aggressive enough and if it failed, radical prostatectomy was not possible due to the obliteration of the surgical dissection planes it caused.

Consequently, I spent the 1980s and '90s in a mainstream urology practice doing large numbers of radical prostatectomies. The cure rate has been nearly one hundred percent and the patients have been some of my most satisfied. I also took a very aggressive approach to good surgical technique to minimize incontinence and sexual side effects. I had patients working on erectile function from four to six weeks after radical prostatectomy. Many men who ultimately would get good erections without any assistance have difficulty from time to time. It has always been my practice to have everyone interested in being sexually active achieving erections within two months of surgery. I have generally started men on Viagra (sildenafil), vacuum erection devices, uretheral suppositories, or penile injections to get erectile function underway while the erectile nerves recover from surgical trauma. Men appreciate this and should expect such care but unfortunately it is not always offered.

Urinary continence also requires determination on the part of both patient and urologist. Many men who will ultimately have perfect continence, initially after prostatectomy, have leakage. This requires aggressive treatment or it will not resolve. Anticholinergic drugs such as oxybutinin–which cause urinary retention–are initially necessary for virtually all post-prostatectomy patients. They all have *urge incontinence* caused by surgical trauma and prolonged indwelling catheterization. In addition, many have *stress incontinence.*

There are two components to post prostatectomy incontinence and, in my experience, most incontinent men have a combination of the two. Damage to the muscular sphincter leads to *stress incontinence* or, in its most severe form, *gravity incontinence.* If the sphincter is weakened, the man loses urine only when he performs maneuvers that result in high abdominal, and thereby bladder pressure (since the bladder is an abdominal organ). These activities are such things as laughing, coughing, or lifting a heavy object to name but a few. When the sphincter is damaged to the point that it creates little or no resistance against the flow of water, the man leaks solely due to the force of gravity. That is to say, anytime he stands, urine will leak out.

The other component of post-prostatectomy incontinence is *urge incontinence.* The cause for this type of incontinence is irritability of the bladder from surgical trauma and inflammation resulting from the indwelling catheter. Following radical prostatectomy, an indwelling catheter is left in the bladder for up to three weeks. This allows the area where the urethra is sutured together to heal. The portion of the urethra that courses through the prostate is removed during radical prostatectomy. This means that the bladder must be sutured to the urethra to restore structural continuity of a urine voiding channel. This sutured area must be allowed to heal before it is ready to have urine pass through it.

The catheter provides the conduit for urine to flow while this healing occurs. Urge incontinence causes urinary frequency and urgency with loss of urine. The treatment is drugs classified as "anticholinergic" which affect the bladder through its nerve supply to reduce the sensation of bladder fullness which causes frequent urination and unwanted, dysfunctional bladder contractions or spasms which in turn cause loss of urine.

Radical prostatectomy is a major operation. It requires anesthesia, post-operative hospitalization and a four to six week period of convalescence. Much has been written about the nerve-sparing radical prostatectomy technique and a number of authors have published potency rates in excess of fifty percent (Quinlan et al., 1991; Walsh, Epstein and Lowe, 1987). Such favorable outcomes are not experienced by many men and significant numbers of urologists believe these published results are overly optimistic. The other major affect on lifestyle caused by radical prostatectomy is urinary incontinence. Many men who do not continue to have constant loss of urine are still bothered by urge or stress incontinence that significantly impair the quality of life.

Another serious issue related to radical prostatectomy is the loss of career productivity and the physical debilitation that accompanies major abdominal surgery. As younger patients with prostate cancer are treated, surgeons are faced with the prospect of taking men out of the productive work force for weeks to months. There are also significant operative and postoperative complications that accompany any major abdominal surgery.

During surgery, patients can have significant blood loss that require blood transfusion. They may experience adverse reactions to anesthetic agents, drugs and gases. Damage to body organs adjacent to the prostate, such as colon, nerves, and large blood vessels, may occur. Postoperatively, such untoward events as infection, wound complications, blood clots, kidney failure and respiratory disorders may complicate patient recovery after radical prostatectomy.

When considering and selecting a treatment for any condition or disease, the equation that physicians use is called a "risk-benefit ratio." The idea is to properly match the risk and cost of a treatment with the potential damage of the disease. One would wish to use the treatment option with the greatest risks for only the most potentially harmful and aggressive disease. When the disease is prostate cancer, there are objective parameters to estimate the aggressiveness of the particular cancer. The two most important of these are the PSA level and Gleason Score. High PSA and Gleason Score of 7 or higher are indicative of aggressive cancers. Gleason 6 or lower cancers with PSA levels of less than 10 are less likely to be aggressive.

Also to be brought into consideration is the low morbidity associated with brachytherapy, cryotherapy, and external beam radiotherapy. All are outpatient therapies–thereby reducing the loss of career productivity to the patient. They all have much lower risk urinary incontinence and impotence, thereby having much less potential of affecting the quality of life.

Many urologists of my generation and our forbearers witnessed the miserable devastation which resulted from late diagnosis of prostate cancer. Our instinct is to react by recommending radical prostatectomy to any man diagnosed with cancer prior to age 70. While this will most definitely maximize survival, it leads to overtreatment of many men who would never have been diagnosed without PSA testing and who would never have developed clinically apparent prostate cancer. This is not to discount the importance of PSA testing in men's preventative health care. PSA testing has led to prostate cancer becoming a treatable and curable disease.

RECONSIDERING THE DIAGNOSTIC PARADIGM

Using PSA for early detection, a high percentage of prostate cancers are now curable. In going forward, we should endeavor to continue maximizing cure and minimizing lifestyle and economic impact. To accomplish these ends, focus should be on making the earliest possible diagnosis when cancer is low in volume and organ confined. Using the Partin tables, it can be determined that making a prostate cancer diagnosis when the PSA is low means that the disease is still organ confined (Partin et al., 1997). If a cancer is low volume and organ-confined, it should be curable with less invasive therapy than a radical prostatectomy.

Patients and physicians cannot control the aggressiveness of the particular cancer, as estimated by the Gleason grade, but they can to some extent control the level of PSA at the time of diagnosis. The lower the PSA, in general, the higher the chance that the cancer is confined to the prostate and the lower volume it occupies. The goal is to make the cancer diagnosis with PSA being the lowest possible–and to try and make a diagnosis before the level falls outside the normal range. Accomplishing this goal means obtaining frequent PSA's, starting at an earlier age, and paying close attention to the PSA-velocity curve for each individual. Practically speaking, this means establishing a baseline value when a man is in his mid-30s. If this level is less than 1, then annual testing should begin at age 40. Biopsies should be done if there is a change of greater than 0.75 ng/mL over the prior year. This should allow diagnosis at a time when disease is organ confined and small volume.

THE GAY PATIENT WITH PROSTATE CANCER

My most recent practice experience has been in a solo private practice which caters to gay men. My patients know that I am gay. Many are referred to me from primary care physicians who inform them of my sexual orientation. Others may assume that I am gay from my staff, who are entirely male by design. Most of my patients are accustomed to talking with gay physicians and are thus generally comfortable with discussions about sexuality. I try to create a sympathetic and supportive environment in which men may discuss any urological concerns. In other words, the patients are not faced with a urologist whose only reference to sexuality is vaginal intercourse.

Like many patients of the twenty-first century, gay men are knowledgeable, and sophisticated consumers in the health care market. They bring information to the doctor-patient relationship and to the discussion about therapy. For the most part, the gay men I treat are like their heterosexual counterparts: their considerations in the risk-benefit ratio are principally likelihood of efficacy, erectile dysfunction, and urinary incontinence.

Gay men may be influenced in their treatment choices by their culture which, in my experience, tends to be more youth and sex oriented. This fact makes incontinence and impotence more unacceptable. Men who desire to retain as much youthful sex appeal are less likely to tolerate those side effects which are more common with surgery. Though radiation may have erectile and continence side effects, the likelihood is less than for radical prostatectomy. There is loss of economic productivity that is generally more significant with the radical prostatectomy compared to radiation options. Following radical prostatectomy there is hospitalization, followed by a period of wearing an indwelling bladder catheter, and a four to six-week period of activity limitation. These consequences may be more difficult for a gay man who may lack the support of a traditional family structure and may have to depend solely on himself economically and socially. Additionally, some gay men may find that their relationships are at risk if they are less intact sexually and physically.

I believe that gay men address issues around prostate cancer diagnosis much like their heterosexual counterparts. In both groups, there are some men who view cure as the mission, almost without regard to side effects. They wish to have the treatment which offers the highest cure rate. Almost inevitably, this group desires radical prostatectomy.

The majority of men with prostate cancer have well-defined lifestyle or career/economic needs so that risk of impotency, incontinence, and disability must be weighed against cure rate in the decision about treatment. As noted above, gay men who are concerned about sexual dysfunction and poor bladder control will accept a lower cure rate in exchange for smaller likelihood of diminished quality of life. There are men who are involved actively in dating and perhaps seeking a long term relationship or domestic partner. They often consider impotence and incontinence as insurmountable hurdles toward successfully pursuing and attracting other single gay men. Additionally, many gay men in my practice place a great deal of importance on masturbation. Treatment choices that might threaten one's ability to satisfactorily masturbate would be unacceptable to these men.

SUPPORT ON THE INTERNET FOR GAY MEN

Health care consumers in the twenty-first century get much of their information via the Internet. There are websites for many different medical practices, specialty organizations, and institutions. Also on the Web are thousands of support groups. I founded a support group on one of the major search engines for gay men who are dealing with prostate cancer. This group grew to fifty members within six months. We have achieved an amazing level of participation from all across the United States and we also have a few international members. There are men with a variety of stages of cancer. A number have devastating metastatic disease in the terminal portion of their lives. Their good humor, candor, and interest in helping and supporting the more fortunate members has been inspirational. Often, when I sit down at the computer with my morning coffee and respond to any messages that are from members needing medical advice, I find myself having to wipe away a few tears. It seems to be therapeutic for these extremely ill men to give advice and support to others.

I began the support group because I found that there was a paucity of groups specifically for gay men. Those that existed were primarily in major metropolitan areas. It was important to have open and meaningful discussions about lifestyle issues with a large group representing a cross section of experience. I have heard about too many men, dealing with the diagnosis and treatment of prostate cancer, who are herded through urology practices with very little discussion; they are steered into treatment plans which reflect the preferences of the physicians and which may not take into account the patient's best interest and concern. Many urologists, I have found, do not work to resolve quality of life issues that may result from prostate cancer treatment. In my opinion, this lack of attention to aftercare is particularly suspect in the treatment of gay men by straight urologists who may be more prejudiced than they are willing to acknowledge. It is my desire to make gay men aware that they should not suffer impotence and/or incontinence silently. They need to be advocates for themselves, and to know there are urologists out there who do care about their needs. I understand the value of erectile potency and urinary continence in making a man feel whole again. My interest in starting the Internet group was to share the experience of my practice and thereby create a larger sphere of influence via the Web.

OTHER ISSUES CONCERNING GAY MEN

I have identified several issues that are unique to gay men. One is a need for greater erectile rigidity to function adequately as the active partner ("top") in anal intercourse. An erection adequately rigid for vaginal intercourse may not be firm enough for penetrating anal musculature. Even if there is good erectile activity after cancer treatment, attaining full rigidity for anal penetration may require additional therapy. Some urologists may either not understand or minimize this need.

Second, with the improvement in medical therapy, we are now seeing a large number of HIV infected men diagnosed with prostate cancer. Several factors about the two diseases coexisting are not known. How will the immune deficiency affect the progress of cancer? How will the new HIV treatment drugs affect the longevity of patients? How will the immunodeficiency affect the patient's ability to handle a major surgical complication?

I view HIV infection as I do any other chronic disease; it does not change my opinion about whether to treat the patient. In my practice, I see numerous HIV-positive men with the diagnosis of prostate cancer at young ages, i.e., under age 60. The explanation seems to be that they have primary care physicians who are attuned to issues in men's health. They are getting very early diagnoses based on PSA velocity changes or low elevations of PSA. They seem to tolerate all modalities of therapy as well as their HIV-negative counterparts.

I can infer some generalities about the care that men are receiving from those with whom I interact in my practice and with my cyber patients. My impression is that gay men are more amenable to aggressive diagnostic efforts. They understand the potential damages prostate cancer can cause and are willing to undergo inconvenient and uncomfortable tests and procedures to give them the best chance of cure. Like the general population, however, I find that they allow themselves to be somewhat too dependent upon physicians to steer them with respect to both diagnostic tests and treatment.

Men need to take responsibility for their own health care and maintain a file of their own PSA values. A number of unfavorable outcomes that our support group members have suffered are the results of being overly dependent upon and trusting the advice of physicians. These suboptimal outcomes are the result of both under and over treating different individuals. Men with ingressive cancers, as determined by Gleason scores of less than 7, and low PSA values, reflecting lower volume disease, are getting radical prostatectomies. I would argue that this is overtreatment since, before PSA was available, many of these men might never have progressed to clinically apparent prostate cancer. These men are ideal candidates for less invasive treatment which has much less chance of lifestyle impediments and a very good rate of cure for small volume, ingressive cancer.

Others are having delays in diagnosing aggressive cancers. Men with suspicious PSA levels should have immediate biopsies. If these are benign, they should still be followed every few months, and there should be continued observation of the PSA trends. If the value continues to rise, additional biopsies should be obtained. Some men get the idea that because they have one set of prostate biopsies that are benign, that this means they need no further follow up. Any man with a suspicious PSA value should be carefully followed by a urologist.

REFERENCES

Carter, H.B., Pearson, J.D., Waclawiw, Z., Metter, E.J., Chan, D.W. & Guess, H.A., (1995), Prostate-specific antigen variability in men without prostate cancer: Effect of sampling interval on prostate-specific antigen velocity. *Urology*, 45: 591.

Oesterling, J.E., Cooner, Wh.H., Jacobsen, S.J., Guess, H.A. & Lieber, M.M. (1993), Influence of patient age on the serum PSA concentration. An important clinical observation. *Urol. Clin. North Amer.*, 20: 671.

Partin, A.W., Kattan, M.W., Subong, M.S., Walsh, P.C., Wojno, K.J., Osterling, J.E., Scardino, P.T. & Pearson, J.D. (1997), Combination of prostate-specific localized prostate cancer: A multi-institutional update. *JAMA*, 277: 1445-1451.

Quinlan, D.M., Epstein, J.I., Carter, B. & Walsh, P.C. (1991), Sexual function following radical prostatectomy: Influence of preservation of neurovascular bundles. *J. Urol.*, 145: 998-1002.

Schroder, F.H., van der Cruijsen-Koeter, I., deKoning, H.J., Vis, A.N., Hoedemaeker, R.F. & Krause, R. (2000), Prostate cancer detection at low prostate specific antigen. *J. Urol.*, 163: 806.

Walsh, P.C. & Doker, P.F. (1982), Impotence following radical prostatectomy: Insight into etiology and prevention. *J. Urol.*, 128: 492-497.

Walsh, P.C., Epstein, J.I. & Lowe, F.C. (1987), Potency following radical prostatectomy with wide unilateral excision of the neurovascular bundle. *J. Urol.*, 138: 823-827.

Whitmore, W.F., Jr. (1984), Natural history and staging of prostate cancer. *Urol. Clin. North Amer.*, 11: 205-220.

Whitmore, W.F., Jr., Warner, T.A. & Thompson, I.M., Jr. (1991), Expectant management of localized prostate cancer. *Cancer*, 67: 1091-1096.

The Ups and Downs of Gay Sex
After Prostate Cancer Treatment

Stephen E. Goldstone, MD

SUMMARY. Although, the diagnosis of prostate cancer is devastating, the disease is highly treatable. Treatment, however, does have side effects that can drastically affect sexual function–both from a physiologic and psychological standpoint. This problem can be particularly difficult for gay men to deal with as many are too afraid or embarrassed to discuss altered sexual function with their physicians and sexual partners. Physicians may incorrectly assume that an unmarried male patient is not sexually active when he may, in fact, be very sexually active. Sexual dysfunction after prostate cancer treatment can include impotence or a weak erection, failure to ejaculate and anal discomfort. Radiation therapy may produce impotence that is of gradual onset often beginning after treatment has terminated. Surgery can produce impotence immediately after the operation that can gradually improve over time. External beam radiation can also affect a gay man's ability to have anal sex because of bleeding, diarrhea and discomfort.

Younger men, men with less extensive prostate cancer and those who have had an active sex life before developing prostate cancer are less likely to experience difficulties with sexual function after cancer treatment. This article discusses treatment options for sexual dysfunction including medication, sexual aids, and surgery to restore erections. Communication between sexual partners and physicians is also crucial

Stephen E. Goldstone is Associate Clinical Professor of Surgery, Mt. Sinai School of Medicine, New York, NY.

[Haworth co-indexing entry note]: "The Ups and Downs of Gay Sex After Prostate Cancer Treatment." Goldstone, Stephen E. Co-published simultaneously in *Journal of Gay & Lesbian Psychotherapy* (The Haworth Medical Press, an imprint of The Haworth Press, Inc.) Vol. 9, No. 1/2, 2005, pp. 43-55; and: *A Gay Man's Guide to Prostate Cancer* (ed: Gerald Perlman, and Jack Drescher) The Haworth Medical Press, an imprint of The Haworth Press, Inc., 2005, pp. 43-55. Single or multiple copies of this article are available for a fee from The Haworth Document Delivery Service [1-800-HAWORTH, 9:00 a.m. - 5:00 p.m. (EST). E-mail address: docdelivery@haworthpress.com].

Digital Object Identifier: 10.1300/J236v09n01_04

for dealing with alterations of sexual function. Sex with another man did not cause the prostate cancer and it will not cause it to return. *[Article copies available for a fee from The Haworth Document Delivery Service: 1-800-HAWORTH. E-mail address: <docdelivery@haworthpress.com> Website: <http://www.HaworthPress.com> © 2005 by The Haworth Press, Inc. All rights reserved.]*

KEYWORDS. Anal sex, cancer, ejaculation, erection, gay, homosexuality, impotence, leuprolide, masturbation, potency, proctitis, prostate gland, prostatectomy, radiation therapy, semen, sex, sexual function, sildenafil, tadalafil, vardenafil

As soon as the doctor says those frightening words, "You've got prostate cancer," it becomes impossible to focus on anything else. A man's heart begins to race; he may feel like running from the room as the floor feels like it is slipping away beneath him. If he is lucky enough to have a partner or loved one by his side, he may squeeze that person's hand to keep away the feeling that his world is ending. He wants to live–that is the plain and simple truth and he will do whatever it takes to beat this disease. Most often the doctor will talk about "treatment options" and the focus is on the big picture of what will give him the best chance for a cure. The man probably will not think about sex because there are too many other things on his mind. His partner might think about sex, but he will not voice his concerns fearing that he will sound too petty or too self involved when his partner's life is at stake. Hopefully the doctor will discuss sex, but he might couch everything in medical terminology making it difficult to understand. And besides, one rarely hears anything else that is said after the word "cancer."

And then treatment ends. The man may find himself lying in bed, thankful that he got through it. Maybe a hand reaches out to touch him or the usual quick kiss goodnight lingers. His heart may begin to race once again; his breathing may quicken, not from sexual excitement but from something else: sexual terror. Sex after treatment for prostate cancer might be the scariest issue a man has to face after the diagnosis itself.

"Will I be able to have sex again?" is not an easy question for a physician to answer because it depends on a multitude of factors. Hopefully one's doctor will have raised the issue before treatment–even if the patient did not. But still, discussing sex with one's doctor early on may not offer much solace when trying to "get it up" that first time after treatment for prostate cancer has occurred.

Before discussing sexual function further, it is important to point out some simple, basic facts that may help predict sexual function after surgery.

1. The older one is at the time treatment begins, the greater the chance there will be problems with sexual function.
2. If a man did not have problems with sexual function before treatment, he is less likely to have problems after.
3. The more advanced one's prostate cancer, the greater the chance one will experience sexual dysfunction.
4. If a man's doctor advises Lupron (leuprolide acetate) or any hormone therapy to combat the cancer, he will most certainly have problems with sexual function. Lupron blocks the action of testosterone and thus decreases libido and potency.
5. Having an understanding partner helps in preserving or restoring sexual function.

Treatment for prostate cancer affects sexual function for two important reasons: The prostate contributes the bulk of the fluid that makes up semen (Milsten and Slowinski, 1999); so depending on which of the two major treatments for prostate cancer a man chooses, he may discover that he has little to no ejaculate at all after treatment. Second, the nerves that stimulate the penis to become erect run close-by the prostate gland (Mulcahy, 2001). They too can be affected by cancer treatment. In addition, anal sex, which may be an integral part of a gay man's sex life, may also be affected by certain treatments for prostate cancer. Sexual function can depend greatly on whether or not the treatment was surgery or radiation therapy. It is best to discuss the various issues specific to each treatment.

RADICAL PROSTATECTOMY

Surgical treatment for prostate cancer is called a "radical prostatectomy." As has been discussed in greater detail elsewhere in this volume (Santillo and Lowe, 2005), the surgery removes the entire prostate gland and some surrounding tissue. The larger the tumor and the more it has spread, i.e., the stage, will determine how much additional tissue needs to be removed. The doctor tries to spare the nerves that stimulate an erection, but sometimes nerve injury cannot be avoided as the surgeon tries primarily to cure the cancer (Jelsing, 1999). Most men notice significant change in erections even after what is called "nerve sparing" surgery. As one urologist likes to put it, "It is more like a 'soft on' rather than a 'hard on.'[1] It is not uncommon to have post operation erectile problems that do improve with time. It can take as long as two years for erections to stabilize. The important thing for the patient is to not get discouraged and to discuss these problems with his doctor.

The other universal complication after radical prostatectomy surgery is failure to ejaculate. When the surgeon removes a man's prostate, the muscle that closes his bladder allowing his ejaculate to move out of his penis rather than back into his bladder is destroyed. Instead of shooting out, his ejaculation becomes "retrograde" and shoots into his bladder. While still perfectly capable of experiencing an orgasm, no ejaculate comes out. This can be a very troubling complication of surgery for some men and their sexual partners. Some men feel that they are not really sexually satisfied if nothing comes out. They may also feel less manly. Semen itself is erotic for many gay men. They like to see it, feel it and taste it. Retrograde ejaculation can rob them of this very important stimulant.

Fortunately, radical prostate surgery does not affect the anus or rectum. Once the patient gets over the pain from surgery and the incision fully heals, he will be able to have anal sex again without restriction. *Anal sex did not cause the prostate cancer nor will it cause it to come back.*

RADIATION THERAPY

Radiation, which is also described elsewhere in this volume (Santillo and Lowe, 2005), can be given either as external beam in which the machine is positioned outside the body or through radioactive seeds implanted directly into the prostate gland (brachytherapy). Like surgery, radiation does affect sexual function in some very important ways.

Radiation works by destroying the cancer cells and–to some extent–the normal tissue around it. The effects of radiation to the surrounding tissue can increase with time, and this is the major difference from surgery. With surgery the likelihood is that a man will have sexual dysfunction immediately after surgery, but it will hopefully improve with time. Radiation, however, can allow a man to have normal erections during and immediately after treatment that can weaken or disappear with time. Gradual onset of impotence can begin weeks to years after radiation therapy and the severity can vary from just a softer erection to complete impotence. But as one radiation oncologist likes to advise, "Use it or lose it."[2] It is generally acknowledged that if one maintains an active sex life, one is less likely to develop impotence after radiation treatments.

As mentioned, radiation also gradually destroys the prostate gland. This can lead to a diminished amount of ejaculate (semen). One may notice a smaller and smaller "load" shoot out and this can be troubling for the many reasons outlined above. A man can still have an orgasm, but he may feel less masculine because so little comes out.

A gay man's ability to have anal sex after radiation therapy may depend on the type of radiation he receives. External beam radiation travels through the prostate and can penetrate the rectum behind it. Seed implants are deposited directly into the prostate and therefore do not have to travel as far. As such, the radiation does not penetrate into the rectum. When radiation hits the rectum it may cause severe irritation, diarrhea, and even rectal bleeding. This can make the rectum sore and anal sex uncomfortable. Fortunately, there are medications that can help. Steroid enemas and anti diarrhea drugs such as proctofoam (hydrocortisone acetate 1% and pramoxine hydrochloride 1%), and cortaide enemas help combat radiation side effects. After radiation ends, symptoms should subside making anal sex once again possible. On rare occasions, however, the rectal irritation may persist and the patient can experience bloody diarrhea. If that is the case, anal sex will probably not be possible. Although seed implants do not usually affect the rectum, they can do so on occasion. In any event, one should refrain from anal sex while the seeds are active; most doctors advise waiting at least one month after implantation before resuming close intimate contact and six weeks before having receptive anal sex.

TAKING ACTION

Communication with one's doctor and partner, if there is one, is critical. Many times gay men are embarrassed to speak with their physicians about sexual function. Most gay men have been taught that gay sexuality is an aberration; it follows then that they might feel that they have no justification to discuss their sexual concerns with their doctors (Goldstone, 1999). This is a wrong way to approach one's treatment. Even if a gay man's doctor is uncomfortable speaking about gay sex (and most will be), the issue needs to be raised. Some doctors will readily answer questions without the homophobia that is often feared by gay men. If one has a partner, it is always best to bring him along for frank discussions about sexual function for very important reasons. A partner needs to hear what the doctor says so that he can better understand what his significant other is going through. His presence will also help "break the ice" by signaling the doctor that this is a same sex relationship. If one does not have a partner and lists himself as "unmarried" on the typical medical office patient information form, the doctor may incorrectly assume that the patient does not have sex. Hopefully, as physicians become more enlightened, they will not make this incorrect assumption and will ask even "unmarried" patients whether or not they have sex.

Impotence, whether in the form of a weaker erection or no erection at all, can be devastating. Men are taught that their erection is a symbol of their masculinity–no erection means no masculinity. Men also are taught that "performance" is vital and most men do not believe they can "perform" without an erection. Anal sex can present further difficulties because it requires a stronger erection to penetrate a man's anus than would be necessary for vaginal sex. To have anal sex one must first pass the sphincter muscles that keep a sex partner's anus closed. The vagina does not have these muscles. A weaker erection might not get through. Even if an erection starts out strong, the act of trying to enter a partner's anus can force blood from the penis causing the penis to suddenly go limp. Using a condom for protected sex can force blood out of the penis, diminish stimulation and increase chances of sexual dysfunction. Some men find that while they attain a reasonably good erection initially, it does not last long enough for them to climax. No matter what kind of sexual dysfunction a patient may have, there is help.

The most common treatment for failed or weak erections is Viagra (sildenafil), and now Cialis (tadalafil) and Levitra (vardenafil HCl). Unfortunately, Viagra does not work for everyone. While advertisements make it seem like a wonder drug, some men will not be helped, leaving them feeling like a hopeless case if it does not work. If the Viagra fails, there are other medications as well as the potential for surgery. If a man's erection is strong enough for oral sex, but not anal sex, and he wants to have anal sex that still presents a problem and is a good reason to ask for help. If the doctor cannot listen to complaints about difficulty with anal sex, it is important to find another doctor who can listen and understand. It is a patient's right to speak frankly with his doctor and to expect his doctor to listen and help.

Although most doctors will not recommend it, a cock ring can help with problems maintaining an erection. A cock ring works by tightening around veins at the base of the penis that normally allow blood to leak out of an erection. The ring acts like a tourniquet and keeps the blood inside the erectile tissue in the penis. A cock ring needs to be tight enough to keep the blood in place but not too tight that it is uncomfortable or cannot be removed. Once an orgasm has occurred, it is important to remove the cock ring in order to allow the erection to naturally subside. A rubber cock ring or one with Velcro or snaps that can always be undone is more desirable than the metal ring variety. Cock rings that cannot be unfastened may be too tight to be removed while having an erection. They can then predispose the patient to the dangerous condition of priapism (failure to lose an erection). A cock ring that works best for the individual may be found in any gay themed sex shop. Most sales people in such establishments are very helpful.

Speaking frankly with one's partner is important; whether he is a life partner of many years or a partner of the moment does not matter. Speaking to one's sex partner is crucial for sexual satisfaction. If one is worried that one's erection will not last or be hard enough, it is important to explain this to a sex partner. The patient must work to get past the shame and anxiety of talking about why he is using a cock ring, taking Viagra or needing to inject something into his penis to get hard. Clearly this is easier to do with a long time partner; and it may seem like an impossibility with a casual pick up. However, if someone is worth having sex with, he will hopefully be understanding and helpful.

There are other avenues for help. There are support groups for men who have had prostate cancer and these can be very helpful as one struggles to come to terms with prostate cancer and the complications that arise from treatment. Information about these groups is available through one's physician, local hospitals, or the local gay community center. Many gay men find themselves isolated in small towns where such facilities do not exist. Some of these men have started their own grass roots group and have been surprised to find many other gay men out there with prostate cancer who did not know where to turn (Cornell, 2005).

While erectile dysfunction can often be successfully treated, failure to ejaculate or having diminished ejaculate is not a problem that can be remedied. Again, this is where communication with one's doctor and partner(s) can be vital. A man needs to understand that he is still a man even if nothing shoots out when he comes. While this can seem obvious, it often is not. It is one thing to understand that manhood does not depend on ejaculation, but it is another thing to understand it in one's loins. Gay men may watch porn movies where the actor shoots a load that could fill a small pond and his erection is hard enough to knock down small buildings in his way. This is the antithesis of what the man who has been treated for prostate cancer may see when he looks between his legs: a limp penis and little or no ejaculate when he comes. Furthermore, the porno actor is probably quite young while the man with prostate cancer is probably old enough to be his father–or even his grandfather. If a man places too much value on youth and virility, it can drastically affect his ability to have satisfying sex. Therapy and support groups can help both the prostate cancer patient and his partner come to terms with post procedure sexual function.

If the patient enjoyed being the receptive partner for anal sex and this becomes difficult or problematic, then speaking with his doctor is essential. For gay men, acknowledging to a doctor that they enjoy receptive anal sex can be a very anxiety-provoking discussion. Talking about receptive anal sex can be confused with one's sense of masculinity. Fortunately radiation injury to the rectum often heals with time and, as stated earlier, the doctor can prescribe enemas or suppositories. If bleeding still continues when one attempts anal sex, despite all available treatments, it just might no longer be a viable option.

When first attempting anal sex, it is important that a man use a lot of water-soluble lubricant. Use of lubricants with nonoxynol-9 are discouraged as they are likely to be even more irritating to the rectum. Lubricated condoms may or may not contain nonoxynol-9, so one must read the small print carefully to find out. Perhaps staying away from lubricated condoms altogether is the most advisable thing to do; and besides, there never is enough lubricant on the condom for anal sex anyway.

No matter how badly a gay man may want his partner inside him, the act of trying to enter causes the anal sphincter muscles to close involuntarily. If one is sore from prior cancer treatments, it can make the pain worse and penetration could tear the delicate lining of the anus and rectum. Even if one is experienced at receptive anal sex it might have been sometime since he last had it–often before the cancer treatments began. To make it easier, it is advisable to sit down on one's partner first. That way, penetration is controlled by the man on top; and if it hurts he can stay there and wait for his sphincter muscles to relax. It usually takes 30-60 seconds before one feels the muscles loosen and then he can sit the rest of the way down on his partner. Touching one's penis while trying to get the sphincter muscles to relax is contraindicated, as that will cause the muscles to tighten further. A better approach is moving up and down on one's partner a few times and then if desired the man can switch to whatever position he likes. This is also an opportunity to discover if one likes being "on top," so to speak. If irritation or some bleeding occurs, he should stop and rest for a day or two. When trying again, experimenting with other positions might make a difference. Some positions will put less stress on the rectum than others and might lead to satisfying anal sex.

If a man has HIV, then it is still necessary to have protected anal sex after prostate cancer. Even if he no longer shoots a full load, or any load for that matter, fluid or reduced ejaculate that comes out can carry HIV and is capable of infecting an HIV-negative partner.

Treatment after prostate cancer can cause the sphincter muscles to tighten if there has been a lot of rectal irritation. The irritation can send the sphincter muscles into spasm–especially if an anal tear (fissure) had developed. Surgery can also predispose one to developing a fissure because the pain medication needed during healing is constipating. Either diarrhea (from radiation) or hard bowel movements (from constipation) can tear the delicate anal lining. Sphincter muscles in spasm are almost as if they are working out at a gym. They tighten and build more muscle mass. When one tries to have anal sex again, it usually feels too tight. If this is the case, a small dildo can really come in handy. Small is the operative word; about the size of one's thumb. To use it, the patient must be relaxed and insert a well lubricated dildo into his anus with constant, gentle pressure. Having an erection while inserting the dildo is fine, but touching the penis is not. Penile stimulation causes the anal sphincter muscles to tighten and makes it even harder to get the dildo in. Once it is in it is safe to masturbate if desired, to see how it feels. If the dildo becomes pleasurable then trying a slightly larger one is recommended. It might take weeks of gradually increasing the size of the dildo to stretch the anus so that it can accommodate a partner's penis. With time hopefully anal sex will be enjoyable again.

Even if anal sex is not possible or maintaining an erection is problematic, it does not mean that all is lost. If a man's rectum cannot be used for sex, it is important for him to remember that he still has a mouth and hands and many other body parts. They can still be used to satisfy both him and his partner. And if for some reason all other treatments fail at helping a man maintain his erection, a penile prosthesis can be inserted. A penile prosthesis is inserted surgically into the erectile tissue. Some types give permanent erections while others have a reservoir buried under the skin that can be used to inflate the erection when desired. It might be surgery, but it can restore one's erection.

It is impossible to expect that the diagnosis and treatment of prostate cancer will not affect a man's sex life whether concerning his sexual behavior and/or what he thinks and feels about it. Fear of sex is very common. A man or his partner might worry that ejaculate can spread the cancer from one person to another. It cannot. Others worry that sex could cause the prostate cancer to come back. It cannot. *Sex did not cause the cancer in the first place and it will not cause it to come back.* Partners of prostate cancer patients often worry that sex causes pain; they often fear that a weaker erection or failure to ejaculate means their partner is not being satisfied. It is important that a worried partner be reassured that what he does gives pleasure and the fact that there is not as much ejaculate as in the old days does not mean that orgasms are not as strong as the ones experienced before the cancer.

Fear, whether real or imagined, can conspire to keep a man and/or his partner from attempting sex. If they have been together for a long time, the desire for each other may not be what it was when they first met. There probably has not been sex during the treatment and recovery period which can stretch from weeks to months. They may feel like they have simply "gotten out of the habit" of having sex. But like the man who fell off the horse and got right back on, that is what is needed. A romantic weekend or perhaps a visual stimulant may be just what is needed to crank up the sexual heat. Communication about fears and worries will help both parties confront the problem, and then they need to do whatever it takes to restore a satisfying sex life.

If a man and his partner were not having sex before prostate cancer and treatment, and especially if the patient was not having sex with anyone, it will be harder to overcome sexual dysfunction. Masturbation is strongly encouraged. The use of sexual aids like dildos, other toys or visual aids can help restore sexual feelings. Even if there is no erection, it can still feel good. A man can reach an orgasm without ever getting hard, and it does not matter if very little shoots out. An orgasm is still an orgasm. If something does come out, there might initially be a little blood in the ejaculate. Though frightening, patients need reassurance that this is a fairly common occurrence but not dangerous. Sex after prostate cancer can be difficult and one may need much more stimulation to get going again. Whether there is a partner in the picture or not, hopefully after the initial difficulties the situation improves as the prostate cancer patient relaxes more and his fears subside. Getting better can take a lot of work and be very frustrating for the patient. With time and trying hopefully the situation will improve.

FOR THE PARTNERS ·

And now an important word for the partners: Communication. If a loved one has been treated for prostate cancer chances are that it has affected the partner as well. Typically, he is worried about what the cancer patient has had to endure; he has offered encouragement to get him through the treatment and worried that he might lose his life partner to this terrible disease. The partner was probably scared but did not voice these fears because he needed to keep up the brave façade. And all through it he probably felt very alone. If he has a monogamous relationship, he too probably has not had sex during the treatment and recovery period and the need for physical intimacy is probably very frustrating.

When the treatment is over he is probably just as scared about touching the patient as the patient is about being touched. Voicing these fears is helpful in getting both parties back on track. It is important to bring up issues with the patient and with the doctor. Patients may not talk to their doctors about sexual problems, but then that is where the partner comes in. The partner can articulate issues that the patient is afraid or too embarrassed to discuss. This is not to suggest going behind his back; but to tell the loved one that there is need for both partners to discuss sexual issues with the doctor at the next office visit. If the patient says that he cannot talk about it, then the partner can offer to bring it up for him. Questions can be written out beforehand so everyone understands exactly what will be asked. That way there are no surprises. Hopefully, as the discussion that has been initiated by the partner unfolds, the patient will join in. It even helps to notify the doctor's office beforehand so a little extra time can be scheduled to speak about personal matters with the doctor and no one will feel rushed. Don't bring up the sensitive issue of sex as an afterthought as the doctor heads toward the exam room door. If a partner does speak to the doctor alone about problems he and the patient may have, specifics about the partner's condition may be avoided for reasons of confidentiality. That does not mean that the doctor cannot listen to what is said and bring it up with the patient at a future visit.

When it actually comes time to initiate sex (and that might be what the partner has to do), it is important to take it slow. Gentle caressing and well-placed kisses can go a long way to quieting fears and letting a partner feel safe in bed. If his penis fails to rise to the occasion, it is not necessarily a sign that something is wrong. The prostate cancer patient can still be aroused even to the point of an orgasm without getting an erection. If the patient seems frustrated, it might be wise for the partner to back off, offer reassurance and then begin again. Asking what makes him feel good and being aware of more subtle cues will allow the partner to know that his loved one is aroused. His erection might be gone, so paying attention to the rhythm of his breathing or soft sounds he makes may be useful cues to sexual excitement and satisfaction. It is also helpful for the partner to guide the patient's hand to his own penis to demonstrate how exciting the experience is. Seeing that the partner can truly be excited by pleasuring him might be enough to reassure the patient that he still is desirable.

A FINAL THOUGHT

Last but not least, gay men are not saints. Hurt feelings and fears of inadequacy, undesirability and even feeling that one is not a man anymore, are natural after treatment for prostate cancer. Just as the doctor provides surgery or radiation therapy to combat the physical aspects of this disease, both patient and partner might also need emotional support. This can come in the form of an understanding lover, a physician not afraid to listen to his patient's fears, a therapist, a social worker or a support group. It must be noted that treating the cancer is not enough; one's doctor can also treat complications such as impotence. But doctors are not mind readers and they will not know there is a problem unless they are informed. Many men are afraid to seek help. Overcoming this fear is essential for attaining a satisfactory sex life. Life has thrown both the man who has prostate cancer and his partner a difficult curve; but with time—and above all love and understanding—they can get through this. Life is definitely worth living.

NOTES

1. Personal communication, Franklin C. Lowe, MD.
2. Personal communication, Michael Stewart, MD.

REFERENCES

Cornell, D. (2005), A Gay Urologist's Changing Views on Prostate Cancer. *J. Gay & Lesbian Psychotherapy.* 9(1/2): 29-41.
Goldstone, S. E. (1999), *The Ins and Outs of Gay Sex: A Medical Handbook for Men.* New York: Dell.
Jelsing, N. (1999), *Prostate Cancer*, Boulder. CO: Westview Press.

Milsten, R. & Slowinski, J. (1999), *The Sexual Male: Problems and Solutions.* New York: Norton.

Mulcahy, J. J. (2001), *Male Sexual Function: A Guide to Clinical Management.* Totowa, NJ: Humana Press.

Santillo, V. M. & Lowe, F. C. (2005), Prostate Cancer and the Gay Male. *J. Gay & Lesbian Psychotherapy.* 9 (1/2): 9-27.

Psychotherapy
with Gay Prostate Cancer Patients

Darryl Mitteldorf, LCSW

SUMMARY. Prostate cancer treatment should run along two parallel tracks: (1) reducing the biological threat of the disease and (2) reducing the psychological symptoms which ensue from internalizing the diagnosis and undergoing physical treatment. Many patients diagnosed with prostate cancer report symptoms of both depression and anxiety. Using examples from his psychotherapy practice, the author depicts and offers treatment strategies for the psychological reactions to diagnosis, treatment, and the consequences of treatment as they affect the gay man struggling with prostate cancer. Prostate cancer in gay men often intersects with the social issues of minority status, discrimination and stigmatization. As gay men navigate the heterosexually biased world of prostate cancer treatment, they must also confront potential problems of stigmatization, including scarring, ejaculation problems, erectile dysfunction, and HIV/AIDS envy. The author stresses the need for gay oriented programs and gender bias free materials as both appropriate and empowering to the community of all prostate cancer patients and their families. *[Article copies available for a fee from The Haworth Document Delivery Service: 1-800-HAWORTH. E-mail address: <docdelivery@haworthpress.com> Website: <http://www.HaworthPress.com> © 2005 by The Haworth Press, Inc. All rights reserved.]*

Darryl Mitteldorf is Founder and Director, Malecare, Inc. He is in private practice specializing in psycho-oncology.

[Haworth co-indexing entry note]: "Psychotherapy with Gay Prostate Cancer Patients." Mitteldorf, Darryl. Co-published simultaneously in *Journal of Gay & Lesbian Psychotherapy* (The Haworth Medical Press, an imprint of The Haworth Press, Inc.) Vol. 9, No. 1/2, 2005, pp. 57-67; and: *A Gay Man's Guide to Prostate Cancer* (ed: Gerald Perlman, and Jack Drescher) The Haworth Medical Press, an imprint of The Haworth Press, Inc., 2005, pp. 57-67. Single or multiple copies of this article are available for a fee from The Haworth Document Delivery Service [1-800-HAWORTH, 9:00 a.m. - 5:00 p.m. (EST). E-mail address: docdelivery@haworthpress.com].

http://www.haworthpress.com/web/JGLP
© 2005 by The Haworth Press, Inc. All rights reserved.
Digital Object Identifier: 10.1300/J236v09n01_05

KEYWORDS. AIDS, antihomosexual bias, anxiety, depression, ejaculation, gay, heterosexism, HIV, homophobia, homosexuality, impotence, incontinence, prostate cancer, psychosocial support, psychotherapy, scarring, stigma, support groups

REACTION TO DIAGNOSIS

Prostate cancer treatment should run along two parallel tracks: (1) reducing the biological threat of the disease and (2) reducing the psychological symptoms which ensue from internalizing the diagnosis and undergoing physical treatment.

In regard to the latter, no one can predict how any man will react to hearing a diagnosis of prostate cancer. The news can come by phone or in person, although, it is usually delivered by the urologist who performed the patient's biopsy. Hearing the words, "You have prostate cancer," can be both terrifying and disorienting. One intuitively knows that nothing will remain as before. One's presumptive world is turned upside down. The affected individual must deal with the physical reality of having cancer and the psychological impact of that knowledge.

Once the diagnosis has been received and understood, a feeling of solitude and aloneness may precede a time of denial. A prostate cancer patient may exhibit a grieving pattern suggested by Kubler-Ross (1969).

In grieving for his prostate gland and the life he took for granted prior to discovering that he had prostate cancer, he may experience denial, anger, bargaining, depression, and acceptance. As in the case of mourning a loved one, this path is not necessarily linear, and one can move back and forth between the various components of this grieving process before arriving at a state of acceptance.

In the author's experience, two divergent psychological responses are typical of men who have been diagnosed with prostate cancer. Some experience a burst of energy and get actively involved in investigating all there is to know about the disease, ostensibly to make informed and considered decisions about treatment issues. Most patients are able to reduce their anxiety by learning more about their cancer and the treatment they can expect to receive: the more direct involvement a man takes in his own treatment, the more likely it is that his anxiety becomes manageable. This may be the case in which the bargaining phase quickly overrides the initial phases of denial (shock) and anger.

Other men, however, may be overcome by a paralyzing period of anxiety or reactive depression. Although anxiety is a normal reaction to cancer, it can interfere with a patient's quality of life and his ability to follow through with cancer therapy. Prostate cancer is usually a slowly progressive disease, so delay of treatment for several weeks is rarely physically dangerous. However, anxiety-based delay can inhibit a man's ability to enjoy his daily life and that alone may be reason enough to help a patient increase his capacity to take action. Anxiety may keep a man from obtaining information, calling his doctor about particular concerns, or finding a referral for a second or third opinion. It may delay obtaining procedures, such as a bone scan or an MRI, necessary to determine the best treatment.

Men who are diagnosed with prostate cancer have reported that their feelings of anxiety fluctuate. For example, each new medical test, procedure or consultation has the probability of triggering profound emotional reactions. A person may experience moderate to severe anxiety, bouts of tearfulness, depression, anger, rage, dizziness or detachment. In some cases, there may be an increase in the use of drugs, alcohol and sex as avoidant responses to feelings triggered by the diagnosis of prostate cancer and the procedures that accompany and/or follow the diagnosis.

Many patients diagnosed with prostate cancer report symptoms of both depression and anxiety. Studies show that anxiety mixed with symptoms of depression often present at a higher prevalence than anxiety alone (Derogatis et al., 1983). The clinician may hear reports of the patient suffering from sleeplessness, excessive daydreaming, lack of concentration and energy, and an inability to perform sexually. Patients may also report a variety of stress-reducing behaviors, such as pacing, talking to one's self or staring into space, that are at once new and disturbing to the patient (Massie and Holland, 1989).

Typically, in the author's experience, patients who have not experienced or been treated for anxiety disorders prior to their cancer diagnosis will not develop an acute anxiety disorder associated with cancer. That is not to say, they do not experience receiving a cancer diagnosis as a psychological trauma. Instead, anxiety may manifest itself in a manner more consistent with their usual coping mechanisms. For example, one patient seeking a consultation shortly after having been diagnosed with prostate cancer announced that he was there only to "gather information." Clearly he could have gotten the information from a book, from his physician, or from the Internet. Instead, he had chosen to come to a therapist's office. While it is often beneficial to provide factual information to the patient, the clinician must not lose sight of the probability that request for facts is likely to be masking an anxiety of which the patient is unaware or uncomfortable expressing.

A patient is likely to become more anxious as cancer spreads or treatment becomes more intense. Thus, another source of anxiety concerning the diagnosis of prostate cancer is learning whether or not one's cancer cells are confined to the prostate, organ-confined, or if the cells have metastasized to other parts of the body. Regardless of the cancer's stage (the size of the tumor and the extent of the spread of the cancer), all treatments for prostate cancer carry significant risks, such as impotence, incontinence, nocturia, rectal bleeding, and others depending on the treatment modality chosen.

The fantasies and realities of side effects are inevitably sources of anxiety. Many of the anxieties related to the diagnosis and treatment of prostate cancer are universal, such as fear of dying or experiencing pain. But other anxieties are relative to the individual's particular bio-psycho-social circumstances. Some men dread the thought of being impotent more so than of being incontinent and vice versa. Some worry about the effects on partners; other are anxious about going it alone. Some men cannot tolerate the experience of knowing that there are cancer cells alive in their body, while others are much less anxious about that and can more easily take a "wait and see" attitude toward the cancer growing within. Each man has both unique and universal concerns that must be explored and processed.

PSYCHOTHERAPEUTIC APPROACHES

In evaluating a patient who presents for psychotherapy after being diagnosed with prostate cancer, it is useful to parse out the pre- and post-diagnosis symptoms. Taking a psychiatric history helps distinguish symptoms which might be primarily reactive responses to the cancer diagnosis from those which the patients might have experienced beforehand. Thus, inquiring about previous traumas, such as separations, job losses, or losses due to death, may be useful in devising a psychotherapeutic strategy with a particular patient. For example, a man predisposed to anxiety may have developed life-long defenses prior to the time he was diagnosed with prostate cancer. Receiving a cancer diagnosis may revive anxiety-inducing thoughts and behaviors which had long been dormant. In such cases, a psychotherapeutic approach might focus on helping the patient adjust to the prostate cancer diagnosis by enabling him to learn more about it while at the same time enlisting his pre-diagnosis adaptive skill sets (Peearlin and Schooler, 1978).

A gay man diagnosed with prostate cancer is often over fifty years old. Having grown up in the pre-Stonewall period, he is likely to have unique concerns regarding any disclosure of his sexuality, his lifestyle, or even talking about his health. However, dealing with prostate cancer will make it necessary to openly discuss all of these issues. For many gay men, these are anxiety-provoking topics which may evoke dissociative responses and avoidance of the subject, even during medical consultations. It is helpful if a therapist can address this anxiety in ways that facilitate the patient's ability to discuss his sexuality, lifestyle and health with his physician and other medical service providers.

It is useful to point out to some patients that they are avoiding full engagement in their work-ups and treatment because they are transferentially responding to their medical caregivers as judgmental, authority figures. On the other hand, a therapist's acknowledgment of a patient's actual experience of treatment providers' antihomosexual and sometimes mechanical attitudes can help the patient either address it directly with the doctor or encourage him to find a new physician. Such forms of engagement can empower an anxious patient. Encouraging the patient's gathering of research data and asking questions of physicians is also empowering. These activities can help a patient move toward a sense of competence and self-mastery. Affirming the patient's information-seeking behavior will increase his confidence in making health care decisions that are ultimately his alone to decide.

Coping resources may mitigate the adverse influence of stressors on physical health. In addition to the patient's internal coping resources, Cobb (1976) suggests that the degree of social support available accounts for the individual variability regarding the affect of a chronic illness upon psychological health. As seen in the following clinical example, psychosocial resources can provide effective relief for patients coping with stressful experiences consequent to their disease (Lazarus and Folkman, 1984).

AB is a sixty-seven-year-old gay man of Chechen descent whose early difficulty in developing relationships led him to develop, in his own words, "a quirky and likeable personality." AB became incontinent as the result of radiation treatment he received for prostate cancer four years earlier. He suffers from symptoms of depression, which include his recent tendency to isolate himself. His anxiety about his incontinence is manifested in his feeling that he "reeks of urine," although no odor is apparent to me when he comes to sessions.

AB's incontinence-inducing anxiety appears to have revived earlier feelings of incompetence and undesirability, which not only are manifestations and a magnification of his depression, but evoke former defenses of withdrawal and avoidance that result in his self-isolation. The belief that he reeks of urine has become his conscious rationalization for avoiding people. His treatment focused on supportive reality testing: telling him that he did not smell, assuring him that he was not alone, and developing a sense of comfort in disclosure of his incontinence thus allowing him to feel more competent and less vulnerable. This process was aided by encouraging him to attend weekly prostate cancer support groups, which he did. Because all the group members shared a common concern, AB began to feel that he was not alone. He was better able to relax, to feel safe, and to begin disclosing his worries to others. The group also served as a reality check for him. AB was eventually able to reduce the fantasy driven anxieties of having an offensive smell, thus allowing him to explore his underlying fears concerning the problems of intimacy associated with being an incontinent gay man.

STIGMA

Some gay men with prostate cancer are stressed by challenges to the coping skills they normally use to counter antihomosexual attitudes such as homophobia and heterosexism. In other words, prostate cancer in gay men often intersects with the social issues of minority status, discrimination and stigmatization.

In the first few years after diagnosis and treatment, prostate cancer may cause a gay man to feel he is set apart from society. To varying degrees, each man feels his self as altered (Cashdan, 1988). If he developed a stigmatized and flawed internalized sense of self as a gay men, he may now have to make sense of yet another stigmatized identity: that of "cancer patient." Some men come to think of themselves as survivors, others as cancer victims. Some may feel greater isolation exacerbated by the new identity of "prostate cancer patient." On the other hand, some men may begin to find themselves having a new, positive sense of self, that having had to deal with their prostate cancer has given their lives new meaning.

For some men, coming out as a cancer patient has distinct parallels to coming out as a gay man. A fifty-six-year-old man, CD, reported that coming out as a gay man was easier for him than coming out as a prostate cancer patient. He said he knew what being gay felt like before he told others, but he could not even begin to predict how being a cancer patient might feel to him. CD said he feared other people would experience his emotions through a filtered perception of him as a cancer patient. Thus, if he were feeling sad, people might say it was because of the cancer and his fear of dying; or if he were angry with someone, people would condescend to him rather than actually acknowledge his anger. Whereas coming out as a gay man was fraught with fears of rejection and disapproval, coming out as a prostate cancer patient was for him more about the fear of being dismissed or minimized. The common fear was of his feeling and being seen as defective and the often overriding feelings of shame.

SCARS

CD had been an actor earlier in his life, and now works as an executive chef. Prior to his being diagnosed with prostate cancer, he had spent a great deal of time in the gym. After prostate cancer treatment he reported some relief in now having a "good reason" to be less concerned with physical perfection, nevertheless he chose a combination of external radiation and brachytherapy (seed implants) in order to avoid external scarring.

The author's experience has been that gay men, whether single or in a committed relationship, are more likely than straight men to raise concerns about how their bodies will look after treatment. For example, many gay men have asked if surgical scars will be visible while wearing a bathing suit, a question none of their heterosexual cohorts have ever asked the author. However, this may change in the next decade as straight men become more focused on how they appear.

After surgery, however, no gay man in the author's practice has expressed concerns about having a prominent abdominal scar. Those who do raise the subject in therapy seem to attach a positive meaning to their scar. Some describe it as a badge of courage, a war wound, a sexy icebreaker, or as something to cover-up. EF is a single fifty-five-year-old gay man. His two months of consultations prior to surgery dealt primarily with concrete issues; but he did have concerns about his post-operative body image. Sporting an abdominal scar some time after his radical prostatectomy, he said that he looked forward to going to the beach and having something to talk about. This may represent an adaptive way of coping with a reality that simply cannot change, but which is not life threatening. Nevertheless, it is always worth exploring the meanings, affirmative or denigrating, that a man may make of his surgical scar.

The therapist needs to be tuned into the underlying issues of self-worth, self-image, and self-esteem into which surgical scars can tap.

ERECTION AND EJACULATION

All men, whether straight or gay, have similar concerns and issues regarding impotence. In addition to being symbolic of manhood, erect penises are important indicators of love and desire. However, for gay men, sex play usually involves two erect penises. The man who has been treated for prostate cancer may not be able to achieve an erection in the spontaneous love-filled or erotically-charged way that might have been possible prior to treatment. Straight or gay, men in relationships initially report that their lovers say, "It doesn't matter that you don't have an erection. We will find other ways to make love." However, as time passes, the partners of both gay and straight men often change their attitudes. They may be more open in expressing their disappointment, dissatisfaction and sometimes even disgust with the impotent partner. As with some heterosexual men, some impotent gay men will seek sex outside a long-term relationship. GH, for example, grew tired of hearing his lover complain about his post treatment impotence. He sought emotional relief and sexual satisfaction from an Internet arranged liaison, saying, "I didn't have to explain too much. We used dildos and it was great." Still others may choose to avoid sex altogether.

Another side effect of a radical prostatectomy is the absence of ejaculate. All of the gay men I treated say that they miss the scent and sight of their ejaculate. Straight men, on the other hand, talk about missing the sensation of ejaculating semen during orgasm. Few of the women partners I have seen mention missing semen as part of their love play. However, about half of the gay partners speak with longing of missing their partner's cum.

HETEROSEXISM

For any patient, anxiety interferes with the ability to act and the ability to decide. All men may experience anxiety while undergoing a cancer screening test, waiting for test results, receiving a diagnosis of cancer, undergoing cancer treatment, or anticipating a recurrence of cancer. Anxiety associated with cancer may increase feelings of pain, interfere with one's ability to sleep, cause nausea and vomiting, and interfere with the patient's (and his family's) quality of life.

For gay men, this anxiety may be heightened by having to gather information about prostate cancer from systems embedded in heterosexual structures and assumptions. Many patients have been frustrated in their attempts to find an openly gay urologist. Gay men report that there is usually a presumption that they are heterosexual during their initial urological consultations.

Most support groups present similar aspects of heterosexual bias. As of December, 2004, US-TOO, one of the largest prostate cancer support group organizations in the United States continues to describe its partners group as a "self-help support group for women whose partners, family members or close friends are prostate cancer survivors or have been diagnosed with the disease."[1]

As gay parenting has increasingly become an option, the author advises patients who are financially able, to bank their sperm. Even if they think they are certain they will never have a child, this gives them the option of having a biological child in the future if they change their mind. Given all of the other costly issues involved in prostate cancer treatment, sperm banking seems cost effective. Unfortunately, few sperm banks seem prepared to have gay men as clients. In New York City, the two largest sperm banks only provide heterosexual men's magazines for inspiration. The forms one is asked to fill out only ask about wives and girlfriends. No consideration is given to the needs of same sex male partners or single gay men. Not surprisingly, the only mention of men as sexual partners is for purposes of excluding gay men, as in questions about HIV (Santillo, 2005).

There has been little media attention paid to gay men with prostate cancer. Publicity around prostate cancer certainly has a heterosexual bias. Public service announcements about prostate cancer feature prominent heterosexual role models such as Yankees manager Joe Torre, former New York City mayor Rudolf Guilianni, and famed golfer, Arnold Palmer. The American Cancer Society has featured Harry Belafonte, photographed with his daughter. The feeling conveyed is that if these macho men are open and expressive about prostate cancer, then all men can be open and expressive. One goal of such ads is to reduce the shameful stigma associated with cancer in a way that will encourage people to seek treatment. However, these heterosexual role models never faced the common gay issue of having to disclose a stigmatized sexual identity. The lack of attention by public health officials to the population of gay men with prostate cancer is, in fact, entirely consistent with a heterosexual bias.

HIV/AIDS ENVY

Ironically, some HIV-negative gay men with prostate cancer present with envy of patients who have HIV or AIDS. They note that there is more formal psychosocial support for HIV/AIDS patients. Many organizations, publications and individual clinicians specialize in helping gay men with the psychosocial issues surrounding HIV/AIDS. In contrast to HIV/AIDS support organizations, there is little prostate cancer support for gay men.[2]

In support groups, HIV-negative men may find it hard to talk about their cancer in the company of men with HIV/AIDS. They may experience competition for care and be concerned that their problems are not going to be taken as seriously. One patient complained that his best woman friend could not accept that his cancer diagnosis was as life threatening and frightening to him as the HIV diagnoses of their mutual friends (Jackson, 2005).

FINAL THOUGHTS

There are many areas for research about gay men with prostate cancer that warrant further consideration. One major problem continues to be the extent to which institutionalized and individual antihomosexual attitudes affect treatment choices and exacerbate psychological symptoms.

Furthur discussion of issues facing gay men of backgrounds other than European-American would be useful.

Meanwhile there are steps that clinicians can take today to better help gay men with prostate cancer. Clinicians can examine their own interventions from the perspective of a gay man presenting with prostate cancer. It would take little effort to read through materials, looking for gender bias. A more difficult problem is changing the presentations and attitudes of many prostate cancer support organizations. But other groups are emerging that demonstrate the viability of gay-oriented programs and gender bias-free materials as both appropriate and empowering to the community of all prostate cancer patients and their families.

NOTES

1. Despite having written to their leadership about this on a yearly basis since 1999, and after having conversed with two executive directors during this time period, their policy remains unchanged. I was told that other than me, no one has ever presented "heterosexual bias" as a problem.

2. Patients with the dual diagnosis of AIDS and prostate cancer have told me that they fear they will die sooner from prostate cancer than from AIDS. But they also seem better prepared to confront the medical world than the men who have not had to deal with HIV/AIDS.

REFERENCES

Cashdan, S. (1988), *Object Relations Therapy: Using the Relationship.* New York: Norton.

Cobb, S. (1976), Social support as a moderator of life stress. *Psychosomatic Med.,* 38:300-314.

Derogatis, L.R., Morrow, G.R., Fetting, J., Penman, D., Piasetsky, S., Schmale, A.M., Henrichs, M. & Carnicke, C.I.M. (1983), The prevalence of psychiatric disorders among cancer patients. *JAMA,* 249:751-757.

Jackson, L. (2005), Surviving yet another challenge. *J. Gay & Lesbian Psychotherapy,* 9(1/2):101-107.

Kubler-Ross, E. (1969), *On Death and Dying.* New York: MacMillan.

Lazarus, R.S. & Folkman, S. (1984), *Stress, Appraisal and Coping.* New York: Springer.

Massie, M.J. & Holland, J.C. (1989), Overview of normal reactions and prevalence of psychiatric disorders. In: *Handbook of Psycho-Oncology: Psychological Care of the Patient with Cancer,* eds., J.S. Holland & J.H. Rowland. New York: Oxford University Press.

Peearlin, L.I. & Schooler, C. (1978), The structure of coping. *J. Health & Social Behavior,* 19:2-21.

Santillo, V.M. (2005), Prostate cancer and the gay male. *J. Gay & Lesbian Psychotherapy,* 9(1/2):155-170.

Prostate Cancer, The Group, and Me

Gerald Perlman, PhD

SUMMARY. The paper discusses a psychologist's experience of being diagnosed with prostate cancer and recounts what it is like for a gay man negotiating the heterosexually assumptive medical world. The paper goes on to relate the author's transition from self-help group participant to facilitator of a gay men's prostate cancer support group. The dynamics and concerns of gay men with prostate cancer within the context of a self-help group are described. Among the topics covered in such groups are gay identities, sexual behaviors and attitudes, feelings of helplessness, anger and loss, HIV/AIDS considerations, partner issues and adaptation. *[Article copies available for a fee from The Haworth Document Delivery Service: 1-800-HAWORTH. E-mail address: <docdelivery@haworthpress.com> Website: <http://www.HaworthPress.com> © 2005 by The Haworth Press, Inc. All rights reserved.]*

KEYWORDS. AIDS, Gay men, group therapy, HIV, homosexuality, prostate cancer, quality of life, self-help, side-effects, sex, support group, treatment

Gerald Perlman is Former Director of Psychology Internship Training, Manhattan Psychiatric Center.

[Haworth co-indexing entry note]: "Prostate Cancer, The Group, and Me." Perlman, Gerald. Co-published simultaneously in *Journal of Gay & Lesbian Psychotherapy* (The Haworth Medical Press, an imprint of The Haworth Press, Inc.) Vol. 9, No. 1/2, 2005, pp. 69-90; and: *A Gay Man's Guide to Prostate Cancer* (ed: Gerald Perlman, and Jack Drescher) The Haworth Medical Press, an imprint of The Haworth Press, Inc., 2005, pp. 69-90. Single or multiple copies of this article are available for a fee from The Haworth Document Delivery Service [1-800-HAWORTH, 9:00 a.m. - 5:00 p.m. (EST). E-mail address: docdelivery@haworthpress.com].

http://www.haworthpress.com/web/JGLP
© 2005 by The Haworth Press, Inc. All rights reserved.
Digital Object Identifier: 10.1300/J236v09n01_06

DIAGNOSIS AND DECISION

I was seated on the other side of the desk from the doctor who, although heterosexual, had been referred to me by my gay internist as a "gay friendly" urologist. It had been two weeks since I had a biopsy of my prostate and I had come for the results. I was chattering away, which is what I do when I am anxious. He looked serious. "I have some bad news for you," he said; then he pushed a piece of paper toward my side of the desk. I remember it said, " Diagnostic Report" in bold red letters. There was also a picture in pink called a "Photomicrograph" with bold blue letters. Then in big red letters I read, "Prostatic Adenocarcinoma." Something about a Gleason Score of 6 (Grades 3+3) and 15% of submitted tissue is involved in Specimen 3. Everything else was in black ink and apparently normal. That was late September, 2000.

My mind went blank. I was in a state of shock and did not want to move. I think the urologist was trying to explain what the pictures and numbers meant, but it was not getting through. He handed me several pamphlets put out by the American Cancer Society (1999) and the American Foundation for Urologic Disease (1998). I recall his saying there were newer versions, but he did not have them. "Something so significant, and you are giving me out of date information?" I thought. He was clearly uncomfortable. He wanted me out of his office, or so it felt to me. He said I should make an appointment with his colleague who was a surgeon. I did not want to leave the office. I did not want to make the appointment with his colleague. I wanted him to tell me that there was probably some mistake, it happens all the time; and I should have another test, or that everything was going to be fine. Something comforting. He mumbled something about PC-SPEC which some of his patients were taking. I could get it over the counter. Then he ushered me out of the office. I knew that once I left his office, it would all become real. I would not be able to deny that at the age of 58, I had prostate cancer.

How had I gotten here? I typically use August to take care of business I have put aside or avoided during the year such as doctors visits. One of the things I had put off was a visit to a urologist. My primary physician had been routinely checking my PSA levels for years. PSA levels, arrived at through a simple blood test, were being touted as the best means of detecting prostate cancer early. And the earlier the better is the prevailing wisdom. Especially for white men over 50. Black men should have PSA levels checked regularly after age 40.

For years my PSA level had been consistently 4.1; just over the 0 - 4 range considered to be within normal limits for men my age (Garnick, 1996; Walsh and Worthington, 2001). My doctor was not particularly concerned about that. So neither was I. But I had been having to get up frequently during the night to urinate; then I would have to wait and concentrate until the stream flowed; even then, not with full force. I figured it was my age. I thought I probably had BHP (benign prostatic hypertrophy): a non-cancerous enlargement of the prostate which is not uncommon in older men and which may cause problems with urination (Oesterling and Moyad, 1996). So, in August, 2000, I decided to see a urologist about this urination problem. As a gay man, I thought I would be more at ease with a gay urologist. I asked my internist, a gay man himself, to recommend a gay urologist. He did not know of any. He recommended the "gay friendly" doctor who practiced in the West Village of New York City. I wondered why there were no known gay urologists practicing in New York City. Were gay physicians afraid to specialize in that field in particular? Was it some form of homophobia or closeting oneself? Was it a public denial of interest in penises? These were questions that crossed my mind as I searched for a gay urologist.[1] So I saw the "gay friendly" urologist to whom I had been recommended. Before I got to see the urologist, the receptionist/nurse had me fill out two universal standardized forms. One form put out by Merck is the "International Prostate Symptom Score" form which asks seven questions regarding urination with responses on a scale from 0 (not at all) to 5 (almost always). There is an eighth question on the form which is rated from 0-6 (delighted to terrible); it is the "quality of life due to urinary symptoms." The latter question becomes a very important question for many men who are diagnosed with prostate cancer (PCa) as well as those who will be dealing with the side effects of many of the treatment procedures available.

The second form, put out by Pfizer, is called the "Sexual Health Inventory for Men." There are five questions about erectile functioning that are scored from 1 to 5 (generally, low/difficult to very high/almost always/not difficult). A score of 21 or less usually indicates erectile dysfunction. The second question got me. It reads, "When you had erections with sexual stimulation how often were erections hard enough for penetration." "Of what?" I mused to myself. The authors of this form are assuming penetration of a vagina–which is a lot easier, most times, to penetrate than an anus. The questions were clearly targeted to straight men having vaginal intercourse. What about guys like me? What about anal intercourse? Hard enough to get a blow job?; hard enough to get a hand job?; hard enough with a cock ring? And what about other sex toys? But I was getting ahead of myself with outrage. I told the nurse that I was gay and some of these questions were off the mark for me. I did not know how to respond to them. "Do your best," she said. Nor did the urologist have much to add.

After a discussion of what has been going on in my sex and urinary life, the urologist gave me a digital rectal exam (DRE). He inserted his finger up my rectum with more KY jelly than I had ever before experienced and he probed my prostate gland. I understand that it is supposed to feel like the tip of your nose. After some probing he informed me that he could not tell whether there was anything there or not. He suggested a biopsy. The word terrified me. I told him I was not interested in having one. He suggested I make an appointment anyway. He said I could always change my mind. I made the appointment.

Then I went through many days of anxiety, depression and confusion. I was apparently having an acute stress reaction. A good friend of mine whose husband died of prostate cancer talked me through it. She said the obvious: Knowing is better. If I did not have cancer, what a relief! And if I did, at least it could be caught early and treated. Her husband did not know he had prostate cancer until it was too late. "Go into the fear," she said.

Several years later I read a story about a farmer who complained to Buddha about his children, his wife, his work.

"I can't help you," the Buddha told the farmer. The farmer was outraged.

"You're supposed to be a great teacher," said the farmer.

"All human beings have 83 problems," the Buddha replied. A few problems go away, but soon enough others will arise. So we always have 83 problems."

Upon hearing this, the farmer questioned the relevance of Buddha's teaching. Buddha responded by saying, "My teaching can't help you with the 83 problems, but perhaps it can help with the 84th problem."

To the farmer's inquiry of what that might be. The Buddha said, "The 84th problem is that we don't want to have any problems."

In telling this story, the author (Bayda, 2002) impresses upon us that life is not free of pain or fear. It is important to face our monsters. And that is what I did. I went into the fear, as my friend had suggested, and I faced the monster. And it was a real beast.

Thinking about the biopsy paled in comparison with the distress I felt dealing with the reality of cancer. For days I did nothing. Perhaps, as cliché as it sounds, I was hoping that I would wake up from this nightmare. What were my options? Where do I get information? I read the pamphlets that the urologist had given me. I had read of Mayor Giuliani having brachytherapy (radioactive seed implantation) and hormone treatment. I heard of Joe Torre having a radical prostatectomy. What else was there? What should I do? I searched for books and on the Internet. But the books had titles like, *The Prostate: A Guide for Men and the Women Who Love Them* (Walsh and Worthington, 1995); *Men, Women and Prostate Cancer: A Medical and Psychological Guide for Women and the Men They Love* (Wainrib, Haber and Droller, 2000); *A Family Guide to Diagnosis, Treatment and Survival* (Marks and Moul, 1995); *The Lovin' Ain't Over: The Couples Guide to Better Sex After Prostate Cancer* (Alterowitz and Alterowitz, 1999); and more recently, Howe (2002) has written a book entitled *His Prostate and Me*. You can bet it is not about Bruce and Roger! While the books were generally informative, they left me feeling excluded as a gay man.

Making a decision is the most difficult business. There is no magic, no guarantee and those damned side effects. Rudolph Giuliani (2002) does a fine job of describing his decision making process. I am not sure if it is more so because I am a gay man or just a man period, but losing my erection was not going to happen if I could help it. Most doctors will tell that there are no erections in the grave; but I never worried about dying and would tolerate wearing diapers if I had to. But sex is so much a part of my identity. It is connected to my feeling loved, accepted, and validated. It is related to feeling powerful and free. It is also fun, exciting, and connects me to a past as far back as I can remember. Like many gay boys, I recall feeling different and being sexually precocious with some of my elementary school chums (Sullivan, 1953; Coleman, 1982). Not being able to have an erection, or worse, not being able to be sexually aroused and experience an orgasm seemed intolerable to me at the time; this despite what Walsh and Worthington (2001) refer to as the big three concerns for men diagnosed with prostate cancer in order of importance to them regarding life and quality of life issues: Death, incontinence, and impotence.

A GAY MAN SEEKS SUPPORT

I decided to go the seeding route with Giuliani's radio-oncologist. Having made that decision, after several months of deliberation, was liberating; but I still felt anxious and distraught. I felt the need of a self help group. I called around trying to find a gay men's prostate cancer support group. I called the NYC Gay and Lesbian Center. No help. I called every group claiming to support men with prostate cancer. Finally, I came across an organization called Malecare. I discovered that the founder of the group, Darryl Mitteldorf, a social worker, was a straight man who in addition to running weekly groups for all men struggling with the PCa, ran a monthly group just for gay men. The only one in the country at that time, I believe.[2] Between the weekly general support groups, the monthly gay men's group and individual therapy, I was helped in the processing of what was clearly for me a traumatic stress disorder. For over 18 months I experienced an emotional roller coaster ride–with highs and lows and sometimes a feeling that the bottom had fallen out of my heart, my body, my soul, my very sense of self– as I processed the physical and psychological changes I had experienced since first being diagnosed with prostate cancer. I share many of the issues I have had to deal with and process with the members of the gay men's PCa support group, some of whom have written of their experiences elsewhere in this volume (Harris, 2005; Higgins, 2005; Jackson, 2005; Miller, 2005; Martinez, 2005; Santillo, 2005).

The founder of Malecare, Inc., aware that I was a certified group therapist and a gay man myself, thought it might be more beneficial for the gay men in our group if I were to take his place as group facilitator. I agreed and I have been leading this ongoing, open-ended group since June, 2002.

It is fairly common knowledge that when men experience conflict or troubles in their lives they, more than women, are likely to shut down and withdraw (Markman, Stanley and Blumberg, 2001). Men, in general, tend to bond around common activities like sports, politics, and/or sex; unlike women who bond around emotional and relational issues. It is therefore no surprise (and it has been my experience as both a group leader and a group participant), that much of the discussion in most male support groups of this type is about information gathering, statistics swapping, and defining ways of making decisions and taking action. Nor do I mean to minimize the importance of those sorts of discussions. Yalom (1975) has highlighted the importance of the sharing of information as a basic curative factor in group psychotherapy.

Other healing factors include the installation and maintenance of hope, the awareness of not being unique in one's experience (universality), group cohesiveness, catharsis, and altruism.

Getting men to express their feelings of despair, their sense of aloneness, and their feelings of vulnerability, loss and helplessness is no small task (Addis and Mahalik, 2003). Gay men are no less subject to these constraints than their heterosexual counterparts. The problem is exacerbated when gay men experience themselves as a marginalized subset of a larger group of straight men. Self-help groups, unless specifically established to counter such issues, simply mimic the greater society of which they are a part; there is inevitably the assumption of heterosexuality mentioned earlier which permeates the culture (Bohan, 1996; Herek, 1998; Greene and Croom, 2000). Any mixed group is a microcosm of the society from which it is constructed and therefore subject to the same assumptive world. The need for a group for gay men only was clear. In discussing support groups for HIV+ gay men, Schwartzberg (1994) noted that when marginalized groups form a sense of community, this has a powerful impact for group members including an increase in their sense of pride and an increase in feelings of connectedness to themselves as gay men and to the gay community. Such a group, facilitated by a gay man, would seem to open up degrees of freedom for its members. Rochlin (1982) has written about the therapeutic efficacy of client-patient similarity for gay men and lesbians.

DYNAMICS OF THE GROUP

What is being discussed here is a self-help, supportive group; not a psychotherapy group. Providing a "gay men only" group with a facilitator who is gay and struggling with issues of prostate cancer himself created an atmosphere in which most of the members felt safer, more secure, and more willing to share intimate aspects of their experiences than they had while attending the larger mixed group. The men felt free to gossip, to be flirtatious, to be campy, and to be as open as they could–given the constraints of gender, internalized homophobia, their individual personalities, and the depth of feelings related to having prostate cancer and the accompanying procedures and side effects.

It should be noted that most of the men in the group have had some form of treatment for their PCa: radical prostatectomy (RP), brachytherapy (SI), external beam radiation therapy (EBRT), 3-D conformal radiation (3-D CRT), hormonal therapy (HT) usually in conjunction with another treatment (CHT), watchful waiting (WW), and/or alternative treatment choices.[3] So much of what will be discussed concerning the processing of issues is not only about being diagnosed and having undergone some form of treatment, but the consequences of those decisions as well: Which treatment option is chosen and why? What are the effects of those treatment choices, particularly the quality of life issues? And what sorts of adaptive/coping devices does one use to deal with the physical and psychological changes experienced?

Prior to starting the group as the new facilitator there were several issues I felt needed to be addressed by gay men battling PCa. These were:

- How are gay men treated differently from straight men by the medical profession?
- How do gay men experience the diagnosis, treatment and after effects of treatment differently or similarly to heterosexual men? Do they worry about different issues?
- What are gay men's priorities compared to straight men regarding treatment decisions?
- What impact does the diagnosis and treatment of PCa have on sexual activity, attitudes and desires? Again, is there a difference from straight men?
- What impact does the diagnosis and treatment have on gay relationships? Is it different from what straight men experience?
- How is self-image, self-esteem, and self-constancy changed, if at all, as a result of the diagnosis, treatment, and side effects of treatment? Is it different from straight men?
- How does the treatment, diagnosis and experience of side effects change the life style and quality of life for gay men? And in what way is it different from straight men?
- What goes into a gay man's decision about treatment options?
- What is unique about being gay and struggling with PCa?
- What are the implications for gay men with HIV/AIDS in their dealing with the many aspects of having PCa?

Some of these questions overlap and they were my questions. Some got answered in the course of group discussions, others not. And there were questions that the group members raised over time.

As it is an open-ended group and numbers of men come and go as their needs dictate, we typically begin each group by going round the room and having each man introduce himself and give his vital statistics: name, age, date of diagnosis, PSA number, Gleason score, other tests and findings, current status regarding decision point, treatment choice and date, current physical and psychological experiences.

The first meeting, with me as facilitator, was comprised of nine men besides myself. They ranged in age from 51-70. Two of the original group were African American, the rest were white of varying ethnic backgrounds. Since then, the group has swelled. At times we may have as many as 15 men attending; but on average 9-12 members attend on any particular evening with a core group of 7 to 8 who attend fairly regularly. The range in age has shifted downward to include men in their 30s and 40s which is much younger than one typically finds among men diagnosed with PCa. In fact, one of the men in the group may be the youngest man to be diagnosed and treated for prostate cancer in this country (Santillo, 2005). We may see more and more younger men being diagnosed with PCa as a result of the more sophisticated and easier tools of diagnosis. In addition, public education about prostate cancer may reduce the fear and shame associated with a diagnosis of cancer and particularly a cancer which may potentially affect one's experience of sexuality and masculinity.

Issues Concerning HIV/AIDS and Partners

Approximately one-third of the group reported having a positive HIV/AIDS status. They are all on medication and doing well with regards to controlling that disease. Five members of the group are in long-term relationships (3 years plus); the others are single and not currently living with or involved with another man. Discussions of the pros and cons of being in a relationship versus being single highlighted some of the concerns that emerged over time. Some single men felt relieved not to have a partner. They felt that while it might be comforting to have someone special to go through the traumas associated with PCa, it might create too much pressure to perform. And performance was not just about sexual behavior. They were concerned about having to be "up," concerned that their experience might have untoward impact upon the other, etc. They felt an intimate friend was easier than a lover in these circumstances. The men who are in relationships are divided on this issue. Depending on expectations–and the ability of each to process what it means to be in a relationship where one of the partners has prostate cancer–a partner may be experienced as a help or a hindrance (Higgins, 2005; Parkin and Given, 2005; Santillo, 2005).

Unlike their heterosexual counterparts, after the initial consultation and procedure, most of the partnered men went to their doctors by themselves. They asked their own questions and did their own reading and research. Their partners were not particularly interested in learning a great deal about the disease; nor were they particularly interested in accompanying them to their subsequent doctor appointments. Their partners went to the hospital, took them there and brought them home. In general, partners were concerned and caring; but they did not want to deal with catheters, urine bags, diapers, etc. Nor did the men in the group want their partners to do so. The group members expressed a sense of discomfort and embarrassment. There seemed to be a sense of "I am a big boy, I can handle this myself"; thus, a denial of neediness typical of men. And their partners seemed to be more squeamish about the unpleasant details that often follow treatment than were their female relatives who tended to be more involved in these intimate nurturing details.

Too often, the care givers get lost and have no place to vent and process their experiences. They may feel angry, deprived, scared, confused, guilty (Howe, 2002). This is not unlike many of the partners of men who have struggled with HIV/AIDS (Doty, 1996). To date, we have not had a partners' group; but the usefulness of such a group for gay men seems obvious. Gay partners attending straight partner groups often feel excluded according to reports from partnered men in the group.

The men who have HIV/AIDS compared their experiences of dealing with that diagnosis and treatment to their experiences with PCa. Most felt that dealing with HIV/AIDS was easier on several fronts. First, and most importantly, they found that their HIV/AIDS doctors were, in general, more sensitive to the concerns of gay men, more knowledgeable about gay men and their health issues. Often the physicians themselves were gay, in sharp contrast to the urologists, surgeons and oncologists they saw for diagnosis, consultation and treatment. Several of the men described how they educated their straight doctors and nurses. Some of these professionals were "gay friendly," or had been recommended as such; but even these physicians often did not "get it." For example: One group member reports his urologist saying that having a radical prostatectomy should present no problem concerning the possibility of having children in the future. The patient was able to call his doctor on this assumption. The doctor apologized and came to understand that gay men wanting to have children of their own may want to consider banking their sperm before treatment for PCa is undertaken (Santillo, 2005). It was the experience of most men in the group that few of the professionals had ready answers to their particular concerns; nor did the books, pamphlets and articles they suggested. These experiences made them feel angry, dismissed and irrelevant.

The men with HIV/AIDS reported that despite the greater ease with the medical community, "coming out" regarding their HIV/AIDS status was initially–and still is for some–much more difficult than telling relatives, colleagues and potential boyfriends about having PCa. There seems to be less shame attached to PCa than HIV/AIDS, even though shame has been a factor associated with cancer in general and PCa in particular (Kaufman and Raphael, 1996). Shame regarding the latter became more apparent as the men discussed "coming out" to others about their prostate cancer. They were concerned about whom to tell, when to tell, if to tell. In particular, they worried about how to deal with new sex partners, whether it involved a one night stand or a longer relationship. "Coming out" is a never ending issue for gay people (Coleman, 1982; Drescher, 1998). The fear of revealing one's health status not only raises its own unique anxieties, it may also trigger many of the concerns associated with "coming out" as gay. In both instances, fears of loss, abandonment, dismissal, and often, feelings of anxiety, depression and anger once again emerge.

Anger

Anger is a common feeling expressed by the men in the group. As noted above, anger is a common reaction to the lack of information available pertaining to gay men and prostate cancer: There is an apparent sense of dismissal felt from doctors, as well as writers on the subject. Walsh and Worthingham eventually changed the title of their revised edition from *The Prostate: A Guide for Men and the Women Who Love Them* (1995) to *Dr. Patrick Walsh's Guide to Surviving Prostate Cancer* (2001). Nevertheless, a perusal of the index lists no reference to "gay" or "homosexual." There is a sidebar in the revised edition to "wives, partners, and caretakers." Some progress! But as in so many venues, gay people seem invisible. No wonder there is anger. This anger is expressed toward themselves, toward God, toward parents passing down faulty genes; and again, there is the familiar experience of gay men feeling flawed and punished. Often, a member of the group would refer to himself as "damaged goods." The feelings of self-loathing and internalized homophobia seem to be exacerbated in the context of processing the experience of having prostate cancer.

Additional anger is aimed at physicians for not revealing certain detailed information regarding possible procedure outcomes, or for leading patients to believe that everything would be fine within a relatively short period after treatment. They would hear their doctors speak of "subtle but insignificant changes" following treatment. However, that seems not to be the case for the men in the group. Their changes have been significant and far from subtle. Understandably, doctors seem to care primarily about saving lives while quality of life is of lesser importance to them. However those priorities are seldom the case for the gay men in our group.

For example, not one of the group members who had undergone radical prostatectomy (RP) had been told that after that treatment, their penises would likely diminish in size. Similarly, no one in the group was informed that after radiation treatment, there was a strong possibility that the rectum and anus would shrink. For gay men these changes can be of great psychological importance. About two-thirds of the group identified themselves as being primarily "bottoms." The other one-third self identified as being either "tops" or "versatile." These distinctions proved to be quite significant, not only of one's preferred sexual behaviors, but also in terms of self-identity and thus treatment decisions and post procedure concerns and behaviors.

Identities, Sex, Decisions

Bell and Weinberg (1978) speak about "homosexualities," noting that gay men are as varied in the behaviors and attitudes as are their heterosexual counterparts. It is therefore impossible to speak of a gay identity as if it were a universal phenomenon. As the group explored self-image, self-worth, self-esteem and self-identity, one participant (Miller, 2005) referred to himself as "15% gay," suggesting that being gay was only one aspect and not the primary way in which he viewed himself. This was in sharp contrast to another member of the group (Jackson, 2005) who refers to himself as "85% gay." He identified himself as "gay first and Black second." The core of his life and everything of importance that he does is organized around his being a gay man. He insists that he could live with wearing a diaper if he had to, or any other physical discomfort. However, the idea of not being able to have an erection or not being able to have sex whenever he desired was completely unacceptable to him. Robinson, Moritz and Fund (2002) have found that brachtherapy was the treatment offering the highest probability of maintaining erectile functioning, followed by brachytherapy plus external beam radiation (EBRT) and EBRT alone. Nerve-sparing RP was next, followed by cryotherapy (freezing).

It should be noted that in making treatment choices, there are many variables and risk factors to be considered. Taking all of those factors into consideration, the man identified as 85% gay opted to have radio-active seeding, hoping thus to maximize his chances of maintaining his erectile functioning and at least to have some ejaculate available when he climaxed.

Previously group members took it for granted that when they got sexually excited they would get an erection, have an orgasm and ejaculate. After receiving treatment for prostate cancer, these three aspects of male sexuality could potentially no longer be seen as a gestalt of sexual experience. They might forever be experienced as three separate parts of the whole where not all three aspects functioned equally well.

The group processed what it would be like for them, and indeed for some it is currently a reality, to be able to experience satisfactory orgasms, yet not be able to ejaculate. Certain procedures and/or medications may render one unable to ejaculate, i.e., one would experience a "dry cum." Several men found some humor in this. They joked that now they could fake an orgasm. Someone suggested producing a porno flick entitled, "When Harry Met Sal." Another man, a devout "bottom," said he was not so worried about erections; that was not from whence he derived sexual pleasure. He was more concerned with the possible rectal complications that often accompany radiation therapy. Another self-proclaimed bottom was so concerned about his ability to be receptive to anal penetration, in a counter-phobic reaction he pushed himself to engage in sexual behaviors prematurely and beyond the scope of the sexual repertoire he generally engaged in prior to having undergone radiation treatment. A group member who self identified primarily as a top suddenly found himself wanting to be a bottom. This was not because of erectile dysfunction, but because he found it infuriating that after his RP, he no longer had a prostate gland. He felt deprived not only of the gland and the surrounding tissue, he felt deprived as well of the option of experiencing what it might feel like to have his prostate massaged.

Helplessness and Loss

Once diagnosed with prostate cancer, one's private assumptive world is lost (Davies, 1997). There is a feeling of loss regarding body integrity, sexual freedom, self-esteem, and control over one's life; and with certain treatments come a loss of body parts and functions. One group member spoke of his depression at the loss of control he experienced. Eight years prior to his PCa diagnosis, he had suffered a heart attack. He said that particular experience had been easier for him. He knew what he could do to help himself: exercise more, give up cigarettes, eat a low fat diet, watch his cholesterol and blood pressure, and take certain medications to control certain risk factors. But after his RP what could he do? He noted that he had done all he could in terms of learning about his cancer and coming to a treatment decision. He felt that as empowering. But once the decision was made and treatment was over, he felt helpless. He saw no way to prevent the cancer from possibly returning. And that was in sharp contrast to the measures he felt he could take to prevent a future heart attack.

It is well known that the experience of self-efficacy (Bandura, 1997; Miller and Rollnick, 2002) plays an important role in the processing of traumatic events. When one feels helpless, anxiety, depression, and rage often follow (Seligman, 1975). The men in the group expressed anger at friends, relatives and colleagues who wished to deny or minimize what they were experiencing. After a while, just as non-mourners respond to those who are grieving (Kubler-Ross, 1969), they felt that most outsiders expected them to "get over it." Some colluded with the external pressure; but most got angry and withdrew. Concordantly, many of the men felt less tolerant of the seemingly minor complaints of others. They were angry at having an "old man's disease." Even though the age of the men in the group, as noted above, was skewed toward a younger direction, they felt aged by the experience; as if they had been contaminated by an aging process. "I am not as I was," one man said. Each felt that they would never know the world and their place in it in quite the same way as they had before prostate cancer entered their conscious lives. They would never experience their bodies in the same way either. They would never feel certain that they were totally cured. The individual trauma/disaster was also experienced in the shadow of the global trauma/disaster of 9/11. A period of mourning is a necessary and inescapable part of the process that each member of the group must experience.

At the time of this writing, except for one man who is an eight year veteran, the vast majority of the guys in the group are within approximately 2 years of having being diagnosed. Some of the older men in the group, 70+, have chosen watchful waiting and will probably die of something other than their prostate cancer. But they enjoy the camaraderie of the group. Most of the younger men, 30s to 50s, have selected and undergone some procedure in order to hopefully prolong life. In this particular group, most of the men who have undergone one of the available procedures are struggling with the side effects of those experiences. Perhaps men who are not having troubles do not go to self-help groups; but the statistics suggest that 70% of men treated for prostate cancer will experience some difficulties that effect their quality of life (Garnick, 1996).

Although inconvenient and annoying, the men in the group are dealing humorously and good naturedly with the incontinence that typically accompanies RP. No one in the group has had severe or prolonged incontinence. One group member reported that a gay colleague of his who did have an intractable incontinence problem got into "golden showers" and was quite sought after. "When life serves you lemons . . ."

Several guys who have had some form of radiation therapy have had so-called "late radiation effects." Some have experienced moderate to very painful burning sensations accompanying urination. Still another man has had rectal bleeding. Fortunately for him, he states, he is not a bottom. But it certainly affects his quality of life. It is terrifying to see blood in your underwear and in the toilet. Here is yet another loss of control of a body function. He reported never knowing when a seemingly innocent passing of gas could become an uncontrollable expulsion of blood clots.

GAY MEN AND PROSTATE CANCER

Whether one sees himself as primarily sex driven, as some of our members do, or quite the opposite, the problems confronting gay men with PCa are in many ways similar to those of heterosexual men, but the differences are also glaring. Thus far the following issues have been covered:

- The lack of information in the field specific to gay men; lack of research; heterosexual bias.
- The issue of "coming out" again.
- The experience of feeling like damaged goods again; the latter being exacerbated by having HIV/AIDS.
- The pros and cons of being in a relationship for gay men with PCa.
- The concerns of self-disclosed tops versus self-disclosed bottoms; and the differences between gay men.

- The feelings of loss of control in general, and specifically of body functions, self-image, self-worth, sexual freedom, confidence, spontaneity and the quality of life.

As the group work progressed, specific issues emerged that gay men may more readily be concerned about than straight men. Some men raised concern about the impact of testosterone. Others were concerned about the relevance of the number of sexual partners and the variety of sexual activities in which they engaged. They were also curious about how their diagnosis, treatment and side effects affected their sexual partners both emotionally and physically.

It is well documented that North American men and men from North-western Europe are more prone to PCa than men from Asia, Africa, or Central and South America (Walsh and Worthington, 2001). It is also known that African-American men are twice as likely to die of PCa as Caucasian men (Lewis, 2002a, 2002c). But it is not known if gay men are more or less likely to get PCa than heterosexual or bisexual men. Nor is it known whether or not Black gay men are more at risk than their straight brothers.

The use of testosterone was raised by several men in the group. Some of the men had been using testosterone as adjunctive therapy to their AIDS treatment. Others, whether having HIV/AIDS or not, used the hormone boosts for other medical reasons or for the enhancement of sexual libido, performance or body image. Somewhat disappointing to our members, but very important for them to know is that while testosterone might be good for the brain, it is contra-indicated for men diagnosed with prostate cancer. A study conducted at the University of California, San Francisco, suggested that higher levels of testosterone may reduce risk of cognitive decline, but increases risk of prostate cancer (Lewis, 2002b). Quite emphatically the International Consultation on Prostate Cancer "recommends that men with a history of prostate cancer not be given testosterone supplementation under any circumstances (Carlson, 2003).

The men in the group represent a broad range of sexual experiences. Some report having very little, if any, sex with another man. Others report having sex once a week with the same partner. And several men tell of having sex daily, or more frequently, with a great number of sexual partners. Questions thus emerged regarding the connection of PCa, if any, to the amount of sexual activity or the number of partners one had. There is no conclusive evidence. But one recent study reports curious results. Rosenblatt, Wicklund and Stanford (2001) found a link between a man's risk of developing prostate cancer and the number of female sexual partners he had. Men who had gonorrhea had a slightly increased risk of developing PCa than those who had not had such infections; thus suggesting a viral or bacterial infection as a potential causal agent. They also found that men who had more than 30 female partners in their life were more likely to develop a more aggressive form of PCa. But an interesting note here is that the study failed to find a link between the number of male partners a man had and the risk of developing prostate cancer. We are still in the dark about the link, if any, of the many various sexual activities with partners, or sites of sexual contact (movies, bath houses, jerk off clubs, etc.), or even the connection, if any, of various masturbatory behaviors to the risk of developing of PCa.

In addition to the effect on their gay partners already discussed, some men wanted to know if there was any danger to a finger, a fist, or a penis that was inserted into the anus of man who had received radioactive seeding. There is no apparent danger reported anywhere. But the prevailing wisdom is that precaution should be taken for at least the first 3 months in the same way that one who has had radioactive seeding is advised about being too close for too long to young children and pregnant women.

The impact on masturbatory activity after undergoing some form of procedure for PCa is an ongoing and avid topic of discussion. Most of the group members–whether having many sexual partners or opportunities, or desires to have sex with another man, or those with frequent or multiple partners–do report on the importance of masturbation as part of their sexual life. Frequency varies from man to man, as do reasons for masturbating. For more on feelings about and the effect of PCa treatment on masturbation (see Martinez, 2005).

As one would surmise, a great deal of discussion in the group is about sexual activity. The men talk about ways in which sexual feelings and behaviors have changed following PCa treatment. They relayed how areas that were once felt to be erotic and sensitive to stimulation ceased to be; how "quickies" are more difficult to accomplish, particularly if one needs erectile aids like pills, inserts, injections or pumps. They speak of how visual stimulation does not work as well; tactile stimulation has become much more necessary for sexual stimulation since undergoing PCa treatment (this is typically true as men age in general). They discuss various ways of staying erect if that happens to be problematic. One fellow said that he never left home without his cock ring. On the other hand, he said that he had discovered new areas of erotic pleasure. His nipples, long ignored, played a more significant role in sexual pleasuring and arousal than they had prior to his radical prostatectomy. Other guys describe finding new areas of eroticism; some even describe having better orgasms. The men speak about the use of butt plugs, dildos, and other sex toys. They wonder about when it is safe to use these and will they feel the same as they had prior to treatment. It was discovered that not all gay men are genitally oriented.

An important topic of concern for many guys is when and how to "come out" about one's sexual challenges. For the men with HIV/AIDS, this was a deja vu experience. In addition to sharing some useful ice breaking techniques, what emerges is a new or renewed appreciation of what intimacy means. The members of the group have developed their own intimacy and cohesiveness (Yalom, 1975). Many members have made themselves available to others in group who may be going through rough times. A telephone list was generated so that members could be available to each other no matter when. Many men are beginning to question what sex has been about for them up to this point. They are exploring the defensive (avoidant/substitutive) aspects of some of their sexual behaviors. They are questioning their own value, self-worth, and self-acceptance beyond their experiences of self as sexually desirable objects. They are opening up. They are revealing their intimate selves, and they are talking about feelings.

THE STRUGGLE

As with so many experiences in life, personality plays an important role. Some men can live with uncertainty and may be more comfortable with watchful waiting or alternative options; others want the dreaded beast cancer out of their bodies. For some gay men, sex may be more important than life itself. One fellow I corresponded with on the Internet told me so. He said that he was involved in a small sex club that met several times a month, and that he had no intention of doing anything about his prostate cancer that would interfere with that part of his life. Thus, he had decided to do nothing in regard to his PCa.

For most people life is precious. Some make the decision to give up sex altogether; others are able to minimize the importance of possible sexual side effects. Nevertheless, in the world of uncertainty that exists for those struggling with what course of action to take when once diagnosed with PCa, it seems that each man makes the decision that is right for him.

It is commonly thought that crises in life make or break the individual. Perhaps, this may be true for some, or even many. But what has become increasingly clear from working with this and other groups of men and women is that life crises tend to highlight who one is and how he or she copes. The journey from diagnosis to treatment and beyond may be considered a form of adjustment disorder or trauma syndrome. It takes time to process. It takes a willingness to reach out, and a willingness to reveal oneself and be open. It takes trust and a feeling of safety to be able to open up and discuss many of the topics presented here. Of all the elements described herein, trust and safety seem to be the most essential if any group is going to benefit its members. For gay men, these concerns are understandably magnified. Being in the same boat with others who have gone through in great measure what you have gone through (the many commonalities that gay men share, in addition to the now shared psychological and physiological changes associated with PCa) provides an atmosphere that fosters feelings of trust and safety. It also creates a sense of strength, mastery and cohesiveness. One group member remarked how strong he thought the men in the group are. Whenever he went for a medical consultation, he noted that the straight men were mostly there with their wives who asked all the questions and took all the notes. He stated that so many gay men go alone. "It takes courage," he said. Most of the men in the group are able to experience a sense of efficacy they never knew they had. They marvel at their own ability to cope with and adjust to a new reality.

NOTES

1. Until recently, I did not know of an openly gay urologist. David Cornell, MD, who practices in Atlanta and has written "A Gay Urologist's Changing Views on Prostate Cancer" for this volume, may be the only openly gay urologist in the country.

2. Since writing this article, similar groups have become available in several major cities in the United States.

3. For more information about these treatment options, and others, see other articles in this volume and the reference section.

REFERENCES

Addis, M.E. & Mahalik, J.R. (2003), Men, masculinity, and the contexts of help seeking. *Amer. Psychol.*, 58: 1, 5-14.

Alterowitz, R. (2002), Sex & the single man. *The Prostate Cancer Exchange*, 23: 7, March/April.

Alterowitz, R. & Alterowitz, B. (1999), *The Lovin' Ain't Over: The Couple's Guide to Better Sex After Prostate Cancer*. Westbury, NY: Health Education Literary Publisher.

American Cancer Society & National Comprehensive Cancer Network (1999), *Prostate Cancer Treatment Guidelines for Patients*.

American Foundation for Urologic Diseases (1998), *Prostate Cancer Resource Guide*.

American Psychological Association (2002), Coping with the trauma. *The Independent Practitioner*, Winter, 39.

Bandura, A. (1997), *Self-Efficacy: The Exercise of Control*. New York: W.H. Freeman.

Bayda, E. (2002), Facing Your Monsters. *Body & Soul*, May/June.

Bell, A. & Weinberg, M. (1978), *Homosexualities: A Study of Diversity Among Men and Women*. New York: Simon & Schuster.

Bohan, J.S. (1996), *Psychology and Sexual Orientation*. New York: Routledge.

Carlson, R.H. (2003), Avoid testosterone in PCa patients, experts advise. *Urology Times*, Feb., 1.

Coleman, E. (1982), Developmental stages of the coming out process. *J. Homosexuality*, 7: 31-43.

Davies, M.L. (1997), Shattered assumptions: Time and experience of long-term HIV positivity. *Soc. Sci. and Med.*, 44(5): 561-571.

Doty, M. (1996), *Heaven's Coast*. New York: Harper Collins.

Drescher, J. (1998), *Psychoanalytic Therapy & The Gay Man*. Hillsdale, NJ: Analytic Press.

Garnick, M. (1996), *The Patient's Guide to Prostate Cancer: An Expert's Successful Treatment Strategies and Options*. New York: Penguin Books.

Greene, B. & Croom, G.L., eds. (2000), *Education, Research, and Practice in Lesbian, Gay, Bisexual, and Transgendered Psychology: A Resource Manual*. Thousand Oaks, CA: Sage.

Guiliani, R. (2002), *Leadership*. New York: Hyperion.

Harris, J. (2005), Living with prostate cancer: One gay man's experience. *J. Gay & Lesbian Psychotherapy*, 9(1/2): 109-117.

Herek, G. ed. (1998), *Stigma and Sexual Orientation: Understanding Prejudice Against Lesbians, Gay Men, and Bisexuals*. Thousand Oaks, CA: Sage.

Higgins, G. (2005), A gay man and his partner face his prostate cancer together. *J. Gay & Lesbian Psychotherapy*, 9(1/2): 147-153.

Howe, D.L. (2002), *His Prostate and Me*. Winedale Publishing.

Jackson, L. (2005), Facing yet another challenge. *J. Gay & Lesbian Psychotherapy*, 9(1/2): 101-107.

Kaltenbach, D. (1995), *Prostate Cancer: A Survivor's Guide*. New Port Richey, FL: Seneca House Press.

Kaufman, G. & Raphael, L. (1996), *Coming Out of Shame*. New York: Doubleday.

Kubler-Ross, E. (1969), *On Death and Dying*. New York: MacMillan.

Lewis, J., ed. (2002a), Why do black men have increased risk of prostate cancer? *The Prostate Cancer Exchange*, 22: 8, Jan/Feb.

Lewis, J., ed. (2002b), Testosterone may be good for your brain but not your prostate. *The Prostate Cancer Exchange*, 24:21, June/July.

Lewis, J., ed. (2002c), African Americans and the aftereffects of prostate surgery. *The Prostate Cancer Exchange*, 25:19, Aug/Sept.

Markman, J., Stanely, S.M. & Blulmber, S.L. (2001), *Fighting for Your Marriage*. San Francisco: Jossey-Bass.

Marks, S. & Moul, J. (1995), *Prostate Cancer: A Family Guide to Diagnosis, Treatment and Survival*. Tucson, AZ: Fisher Books.

Martinez, R. (2005), Prostate cancer and sex. *J. Gay & Lesbian Psychotherapy*, 9(1/2): 91-99.

Miller, M. (2005), Identity and prostate cancer: Comments on a messy life. *J. Gay & Lesbian Psychotherapy*, 9(1/2): 119-129.

Miller, W.R. & Rollnick, S. (2002), *Motivational Interviewing: Preparing for Change (Second Edition)*. New York: Guilford Press.

Oesterling, J. & Moyad, M. (1996), *The ABCs of Prostate Cancer: The Book That Can Save Your Life*. Madison House: National Book Network.

Parkin, R. & Girven, H. (2005), Together with prostate cancer. *J. Gay & Lesbian Psychotherapy*, 9(1/2): 137-146.

Robinson, J.W., Moritz, S., & Fung, T. (2002), Meta-analysis of rates of erectile function after treatment of localized prostate carcinoma. *Int. J. Radiation Oncology, Biology, and Physics*, 54(4): 1063-1068.

Rochlin, M. (1982), Sexual orientation of the therapist and effectiveness with gay clients. *J. Homosexuality*, 7: 21-30.

Rosenblatt, K.A., Wicklulnd, K.G. & Stanford, J.L. (2201), Sexual factors and the risk of prostate cancer. *Amer. J. Epid.*, 153(12): 1152-1158.

Santillo, V.M. (2005), Prostate cancer diagnosis and treatment of a 33-year-old gay man. *J. Gay & Lesbian Psychotherapy*, 9(1/2): 155-170.

Schaffner, B. (2005), Prostate cancer at age 84. *J. Gay & Lesbian Psychotherapy*, 9(1/2): 131-136.

Schwartzberg, S.S. (1993), Struggle for meaning: How HIV-positive gay men make sense of AIDS. *Prof. Psychol: Res. and Pract.*, 24(4): 483-490.

Schwartzberg, S.S. (1994), Vitality and growth in HIV-infected gay men. *Soc. Sci. and Med.*, 38(4): 593-602.

Seligman, M.E.P. (1975), *Helplessness: On Depression, Development, and Death*. San Francisco: W.H. Freeman.

Siegel, K. & Meyer, I.H. (1999), Hope and resilience in suicide ideation and behavior of gay and bisexual men following notification of HIV infection. *AIDS Educ. and Prevent.*, 11(1): 53-64.

Sullivan, H.S. (1953), *The Interpersonal Theory of Psychiatry*. New York: Norton.

Wainrib, B., Haber, S. & Droller, M. (1996), *Prostate Cancer: A Guide for Women and the Men They Love*. New York: Dell Publishing Group.

Wallner, K. (1996), *Prostate Cancer: A Non-Surgical Perspective.* Canaan, NY: Smart Medicine Press.

Walsh, P. & Worthington, J. (1995), *The Prostate: A Guide for Men and the Women Who Love Them.* Baltimore: The Johns Hopkins University Press.

Walsh, P. & Worthington, J. (2001), *Dr. Patrick Walsh's Guide to Surviving Prostate.* New York: Warner Books.

Yalom, I. (1975), *The Theory and Practice of Group Psychotherapy (Second Edition).* New York: Basic Books.

FROM THE PERSPECTIVE
OF GAY MEN WITH PROSTATE CANCER

Prostate Cancer and Sex

Roberto Martinez

SUMMARY. A sexually active Latino gay man describes how the surgical removal of his prostate gland affected his thoughts, feelings, attitudes and activities about sexuality in general and specifically about how the physical changes he experienced engendered emotional changes in his own struggles with sex and masturbation. The author focuses on the experience of orgasms without ejaculation, his changing views and experiences of sex, the feelings of aging engendered by a diagnosis of prostate cancer, and his search for support after diagnosis and treatment. *[Article copies available for a fee from The Haworth Document Delivery Service: 1-800-HAWORTH. E-mail address: <docdelivery@haworthpress.com> Website: <http://www.HaworthPress.com> © 2005 by The Haworth Press, Inc. All rights reserved.]*

Roberto Martinez is a doctoral candidate in the Department of Urban Education at the CUNY Graduate Center. A former board memeber of Latino Gay Men of New York, he is currently an advisor at the Steinhardt School of Education at New York University.

[Haworth co-indexing entry note]: "Prostate Cancer and Sex." Martinez, Roberto. Co-published simultaneously in *Journal of Gay & Lesbian Psychotherapy* (The Haworth Medical Press, an imprint of The Haworth Press, Inc.) Vol. 9, No. 1/2, 2005, pp. 91-99; and: *A Gay Man's Guide to Prostate Cancer* (ed: Gerald Perlman, and Jack Drescher) The Haworth Medical Press, an imprint of The Haworth Press, Inc., 2005, pp. 91-99. Single or multiple copies of this article are available for a fee from The Haworth Document Delivery Service [1-800-HAWORTH, 9:00 a.m. - 5:00 p.m. (EST). E-mail address: docdelivery@haworthpress.com].

Digital Object Identifier: 10.1300/J236v09n01_07

KEYWORDS. Aging, cancer, ejaculation, gay, Latino, masturbation, orgasm, prostate, prostatectomy, sex

INTRODUCTION

Two weeks before I turned 40, I had a radical retropubic prostatectomy (RRP) in order to combat prostate cancer (PCa). At the time it was the only choice, for me, a thirty-nine year old Latino gay male with a baseline PSA of 7.9, a Gleason Score of 6 and a strong family history of prostate cancer: one uncle with the disease and a father who died of metastatic prostate cancer four months earlier.

I'd like to say my personal struggle was the most important thing in the world, but at that time my life, and the world, were both in chaos. In brief, a history of that time reads as follows: September the 11th (I work a mile and a half away from ground zero); my father died; I moved to Brooklyn; then I was diagnosed with the same disease that claimed my father. Terrorism and cancer were my companions.

I pondered treatment options. Seed implants were promising but the research data covered only twelve years at most. At the age of thirty-nine, I wanted data that went back far enough to suggest that I might have at least another forty years to live. I read books and surfed the web for alternative treatment options. I dared to be skeptical of surgeons and the so-called "gold standard" of treatment: the surgical removal of the prostate gland. The herbal remedy I sought that would make this all go away did not exist. Even the radiation oncologist with whom I consulted said that he might opt for surgery if he were in my shoes; and he was even younger than me. The treatment for me was clear.

In retrospect the decision to have surgery and the resulting medical recovery were the easy parts. I had a good surgeon. He spared my nerves, so I would probably be able feel sexual excitement and have erections. My margins were good, indicating that the cancer had not spread beyond the capsule of the prostate. Wearing a catheter was a drag, but that lasted only about a week. By the time the catheter was removed, my urinary continence was intact. I was very relieved to be feeling well and not in need of a diaper. I healed rapidly. Three days after leaving the hospital, I was walking up and down the four flights of stairs to my top-floor brownstone flat; within three weeks I was without much pain or discomfort. I felt secure in the knowledge that I had done the right thing for my long-term health. But being a sexually active gay man, the fact that I would never ejaculate again was not something even imaginable until it became all too real.

Prior to my diagnosis of PCa, I had indeed, been a very sexually active man. I first had man to man sex in the late 1970s while in my early teens. I first entered a gay bar in 1978 at the age of sixteen. It was a leather bar in Detroit called the Interchange. Walking into the women's room there and seeing men in various stages of what I then considered depraved and wanton sex, filled me with both erotic desire and moral repulsion; it so conflicted with my Catholic school upbringing. Desire and desperation fueled my teenage sexual drive while, at the same time, I surrounded myself with school and work. I learned to veil the shame I felt about my sex life with attempts at respectability and honor. Any orgies would come much later; but then all was hidden. I would indulge my sexual desires later, through my early 30s. In retrospect, I am glad I did.

In 1982, I fell in love with a man, and painfully realized the common materialist fantasies of having a wife and kids and a home in the suburbs would not be mine. I stayed with my lover for six years, probably longer than I should have, because we were each afraid to be alone with our desires during those first years of the AIDS epidemic. Falling in love saved me; being in Boston and not New York saved me; but mostly being open about my feelings pro and con saved me and gave me the courage to practice safer sex. I was one of the lucky ones. Today, I feel I still am.

Having sex after prostate cancer is a lot like learning to enjoy safer sex. It is not the same, nor is it "the real thing." But if I wanted to enjoy life, if I wanted to have a future sex life, it was something I had to learn to appreciate. Doctors say nerve sparing surgery preserves 60% of the nerve endings, 20% of which will grow back; yet about 20% are damaged forever never to return. Usually, the older the patient, the less robust the nerve endings. As my doctor said, "Is your erection the same as it was when you were 18? Well, sparing the nerves will not give you the erection of a teenager."

ORGASMS WITHOUT EJACULATION

My first post-surgical orgasm was about 3 weeks after surgery. I was not erect. Something the doctors and nurses repeatedly told me throughout the prep and recovery is that men can have an orgasm without an erection and without an ejaculation. Though this seemed obvious to me, as one who had experienced at least a few orgasms without ejaculation, I can honestly say that the idea of having an orgasm without an ejaculation was never once a stated goal of mine. After surgery, however, it was the only option.

I did not know what my life would be like without my own cum, without an ejaculate. Given my sexual history, I never imagined that re-learning how to have an orgasm would ever be a concern of mine. That I would have to relearn how to give myself an orgasm was more of a shock than this boy could take. After more than twenty years of sexual activity, relearning how to masturbate was a frustration, a slap in the face, a nuisance. It made me feel angry and defiant. In some ways re-learning how to masturbate was the hardest thing to learn about life after prostatectomy, and relearning how to masturbate without cum was a special challenge.

A prostatectomy changes how one masturbates. It is that simple. Simple hand to cock stimulation does not always cut it anymore. In fact, for about four months, I barely tried to masturbate, as I was almost afraid my body would disappoint me. One morning before work, horny out of my mind, I finally laid down to beat off without the aid of Viagra (sildenafil) or a cockring. I slowly beat my limp dick until I finally achieved unadulterated release. It worked–that is it relieved stress–but it fell somewhere short of expectations. Before surgery, I would think nothing of taking matters into my own hand should desire overcome me. If a quickie encounter with someone were not possible, then a quick JO would do, releasing tension and strain, and making it possible to get my mind back on work, a mortgage, or my salary. After surgery I learned that this sort of quickie jacking off was not as satisfying.

Masturbation after prostate cancer surgery demanded a total recon-sideration of my erogenous zones because stimulation of my cock and my balls alone often proved to be an exercise in futility. I know from some men, using porn increases excitement; but for me, it often exacer-bated feelings of inadequacy. In my case, touch and fondling of the nip-ples, caressing of my body, help relax and excite me. Self-massage of arms, legs, feet and hands go a long way in soothing my soul and nerves. Stretching of torso and limb had the effect of loosening my daily stresses and strains. Much more than before, sex and even masturbation is now about giving over of my total mind and body, not just my geni-tals, to fulfill a need. Previously, hand-to-cock stimulation alone was enough to light and stoke the fires, but purely genital stimulation now left me wanting. My heart AND mind had to be in it or it was not going to work. Sometimes really good porn helped, but it often made me feel self-conscious. Maybe it was because I had fewer nerve endings in my nether regions. Mostly I was simply more anxious about my sexual per-formance period and this alone played mind games with my sexual functioning. Whether physical or psychological, I had to come up with new techniques and mindsets in order to gain control over my new body. I had to think of new ways to smoke out negativity and focus concentration on the desire to make sexual activity worthwhile again.

Nor can sex with a partner be tied to a kind of check-off list of stimulators that once worked so easily. Time, preparation and foreplay are paramount. Quality body time is key. This is as true in my own masturbation as in sexual relations with a partner. The days of rushing to jerk off to release frustrations are mostly over. Like bad sex, a lousy masturbatory experience is usually not worth the time it takes to shuck your shorts. After prostate cancer, bad masturbation defeated me on multiple levels, reminding me that the plumbing had changed, that I could no longer shoot–often discouraging me from taking matters into my own hands.

There is no cum anymore. The first few months of learning about and getting used to my new body, it was repeatedly shocking to masturbate myself to a pleasant orgasm, for I had no visual cue to affirm my orgasm. Having an orgasm was generally not a visual experience after surgery. Yes, I had the tightening of muscles and balls. Yes, I can have a moment of great release; but now, the amount of work necessary for this sexual experience is greatly increased. Of course I can still cum. I just don't shoot anymore and this is new and permanent.

Sometimes when my orgasm was not that strong, I wondered if I had really cum at all. Had I faked it? Or had I just gotten myself really, really aroused, so much so, that even my little pre-orgasm was almost enough for me? I never imagined before that it could be possible for a man to even fake an orgasm, but given that no ejaculate is present, it is technically possible to fake one's own orgasm. On at least a couple of occasions, I had to be content with just getting really close yet never finishing it off. From my own standpoint, it's not worth the trouble. What is the point of faking your own masturbatory orgasm? Perhaps one's security in this comes with age saying it's OK to just be held and intimate and not cum. Perhaps it is OK to just be aroused and not really shoot. Sometimes it just feels like a premature ejaculation under your own skin. It's as if one came slightly but it was not really satisfying. Premature ejaculation without cum is particularly confounding. I wondered, "Did I come too soon? Did I come at all?"

Anonymous sexual encounters can be great, but they are often fraught with different stresses. On more than a few occasions, I've had a wonderful sexual encounter with a relative stranger only to have my sex partner interject, "Wow, man, you did everything but come!" Ninety percent of the time it is not worth discussing post-coitally; but at other times, I find that sexual intimacy begets a desire for further closeness. On occasion, I've volunteered sheepishly afterward that I was sorry I didn't come. I allowed that I had cancer a few years back, only to have the guy retort, "Wow man, I didn't even notice." Sometimes I feel that men can be such pigs.

Occasionally, I've tried to explain on-line, before we meet, that I had cancer and though I can have an orgasm, I can't ejaculate. That approach usually works only for people I've had some on-line rapport with over time. However, usually in a moment of compelling passion, I find there is seemingly no point in going there. The aim for me is to reach the point of no return in the bedroom, not to reach that point before I connect.

CHANGING VIEWS AND EXPERIENCES OF SEX

A prostatectomy changed how I had sex. I notice now that I have about two or three different kinds of orgasms. I can still have a mind-blowing orgasm and that is absolutely the best news of all. The tensing of all bodily muscles, the mental focus needed to make sex successful; these are all things that happen more frequently with my current domestic partner and no one is happier about that than me. Even a mediocre orgasm can be better than previously because before the surgery, the aim would merely be to bust a nut. Now the aim is not only to bust a nut, but also to convince myself that it is worth the half hour of planning needed for Viagra to kick in, or to wear a cockring, and/or to suppress any fear of performance anxiety I might have. As for a weak orgasm, it is almost not even worth going there at all. I notice that I tend to "save" it a lot more than I used to, but I don't know how much of this is a factor of getting to be more middle-aged and how much of it is the new plumbing.

A prostatectomy changed how I think of sex with my partner. Talking with a steady partner and taking time and planning sex makes a world of difference. If anything, I've noticed that sex with my partner is more valuable for me. Maybe it is because having a steady partner takes some of the guesswork out of negotiating my body. Maybe it's because my partner knows over the long term how best to please and be pleased. Maybe it's because once you have a partner who helps you through cancer you realize what their true mettle is, and that this is more valuable than any orgasm alone.

A prostatectomy changed how I think of women. Mostly in terms of what works for me sexually, the caressing, the touch, the time and the trust, sound vaguely reminiscent to how women often talk about "making love." It is a complete and total body experience, maybe involving evolutionary desires to be protected and procreate. Perhaps that lack of an external indicator of sexual release (cum/ejaculate) makes the concentration of desire a much more worthy goal. Men can always look to a visual frame of reference for physiological completion. For me, after a prostatectomy, it is no longer a simple visual frame of reference that produces knowledge of my own pleasure. It is not something external that validates your claim to an orgasm. Sex for a man after prostate surgery, at least for me, has validity only when it is internally valid. External validation is limited to an erection alone.

PROSTATE CANCER AND AGING

Sex after prostate cancer is implicitly connected with getting older, and at age 39, I definitely had to confront the shock of aging at an earlier age than most of my peers. A friend with prostate cancer, who is even younger than me, said that he felt that he was kicked into instant middle-age with his diagnosis–and he is right of course. I developed some strong connections with men in their sixth and seventh decade of life and now, of course, I had more in common with other men who died in their 70s. I no longer easily discount the feelings of older men. A greater appreciation for older men went hand in hand with my experience with prostate cancer.

My midlife crisis occurred when, at the age of thirty-nine, I realized that I had more in common with the average 60-year-old man than I did with my own peers. I immediately felt this incredible kinship with older men, as they were the only ones who seemed to know what I was talking about. Men's understanding about prostate cancer seemed directly proportional to their ages; the older they were, the greater the level of their understanding. Some younger men had exposure to people in their own families with the disease. However, on the whole, this was not something I expected most men in their 30s to even care about much less know. I think a few men who were in their 20s and to whom I spoke honestly about my cancer seemed almost afraid of me as though I were an old man! Sure I was angry for a while about feeling old, but in the grand scheme of things prostate cancer is a good cancer to have. A great deal is known about how to reduce complications and to extend one's life. And it is a relatively slow moving cancer. After seeing children with cancer in my trips to my oncologist, children who had never lived a life, I knew how lucky I was.

SUPPORT

In the days after my prostatectomy, I went to a gay male prostate cancer support group to help sort out my thoughts, and most days discussions centered on the disease and its cure. But after a relatively short period of time, I was most interested in focusing on the emotional dimensions of my sexual future. Perhaps it was because like many in this community I had a close relative with the disease. That my sexuality was so important to me, made me painfully aware of how my father's experience with prostate cancer must have been. In the months after my surgery, I met many men who had the same consequences with their prostate surgery as my father had. His operation in the late 1980s predated today's nerve-sparing techniques, and he suffered from total impotence for the last 15 years of his life. In the group, men would speak of their own struggles with impotence; and in their anger and frustration I heard my own father speaking to me from a world beyond. How I wish I could have talked to him from my current perspective.

Oh the questions I would ask, or wouldn't ask. My father lacked much formal education and was fatalistic. When he was given his diagnosis of cancer, he said it was if someone had stabbed him in the back. Still in his silence and pain, I would want to know: Did you know you would be impotent before you had surgery? How long did it take for you to come to terms with it? Did you have other friends who went through this with you, or did you keep it to yourself? Did your faith in God help? How did my mother help? How did your former mistress help? Is that why you supported me in front of Mom in my desire to go out at night? Did you want me to know someone could enjoy the fruits of manhood? Still these questions went unasked, unimagined even. My father was a man obsessed with his own mortality. We once traveled throughout Mexico in 1974 because of a dream my father had that he would die that year. My father had been planning for his death for at least 25 years before it happened. When it finally did happen, my siblings all gathered and said, "Well, this is finally it." Little did I know I would think of him every single day for more than a year after my treatment for prostate cancer. My closeness to him in death, made it difficult to be surrounded by men in the same circumstance.

After a couple of months, I could not go to certain meetings because of their emphasis on complex major health problems and my seemingly self-centered focus on my minor surmountable ones. I lived in a new age, the age of Viagra; an age that eerily coincided with the post 9/11 world. I have no ejaculate, but I do have erections, medically induced or enhanced if necessary. So all is not lost. I was witness to the worst of transgressions, but I was not a major victim of it myself. I was prone to be a victim of my own anger and fear but only if I let it. I cannot go back in time, and I cannot spend time contemplating the past. Like the twin towers, my ejaculate was never coming back and pretending it would was self-defeatist. I have smoked out my own Osama and he cannot hunt me down.

Surviving Yet Another Challenge

Lidell Jackson

SUMMARY. Describing himself as a physically fit and sexually-active African-American gay man of mature years, and having survived more than a decade of being HIV-positive, the author writes about being faced with another significant and completely new challenge to his health and quality of life: prostate cancer. He describes his choice of treatment and road to recovery in the context of his own personal philosophy of life. *[Article copies available for a fee from The Haworth Document Delivery Service: 1-800-HAWORTH. E-mail address: <docdelivery@haworthpress.com> Website: <http://www.HaworthPress.com> © 2005 by The Haworth Press, Inc. All rights reserved.]*

KEYWORDS. Assertive self care, African American men, gay, erection, HIV+, libido, men of color, prostate cancer, sex-positive, testosterone

As a former Ballet and Broadway Dancer–and a pretty good Wrestler in turn–I've always prided myself on being both physically healthy and extremely in touch with my physicality. I'm also a longstanding political activist in the LGTSBT (lesbian/gay/two spirit/bisexual/transgender) community. I am also an HIV-positive, sex-positive activist who runs

Lidell Jackson is a former ballet and Broadway dancer. He is a long time gay activist. He holds a BA in applied mathematics from Brown University.

[Haworth co-indexing entry note]: "Surviving Yet Another Challenge." Jackson, Lidell. Co-published simultaneously in *Journal of Gay & Lesbian Psychotherapy* (The Haworth Medical Press, an imprint of The Haworth Press, Inc.) Vol. 9, No. 1/2, 2005, pp. 101-107; and: *A Gay Man's Guide to Prostate Cancer* (ed: Gerald Perlman, and Jack Drescher) The Haworth Medical Press, an imprint of The Haworth Press, Inc., 2005, pp. 101-107. Single or multiple copies of this article are available for a fee from The Haworth Document Delivery Service [1-800-HAWORTH, 9:00 a.m. - 5:00 p.m. (EST). E-mail address: docdelivery@haworthpress.com].

his own safe sex club for "Men Of Color and Their Friends." This represents more than 30 years of an adult life in which I've prided myself on being physically fit. Even as my community has weathered the horrors of an AIDS pandemic–and so many of us have seen so many of our strong, healthy gay male friends and lovers get sick and die–I've still maintained an identity of superior physical health.

During my dance years I discovered homeopathy–the science of treating diseases by administering minute doses of remedies that, in healthy people, produce symptoms of the diseases being treated, thereby causing the body's immune system to actively engage in healing itself. I particularly enjoyed the idea that my discipline and adherence to a strong physical regimen made my body an active, important partner with my homeopath in continuing to keep myself healthy.

Of course, all of this was brought into question when I sero-converted in 1991. For over eight years I was faced with the dilemma of how my reliance upon homeopathy would keep me from progressing to a situation where I developed AIDS. I worked diligently with my homeopath to incorporate blood, colloidal, anti-viral and immune-building natural remedies into my already "hyper-disciplined" pill-taking regimen.

ALTERNATIVE HEALING

The Summer of '99 presented me with my "Lazarus moment." After coordinating and supervising an overwhelmingly stressful camping weekend involving 60-plus gay men, a staff, a caterer, and daily chartered buses and vans, I suddenly developed an especially harrowing case of spinal meningitis–paralysis of my spine. This resulted in three weeks of intense hospitalization, four weeks of very confining home convalescence with hourly injections of Rocephin through a Hickman catheter in my chest, and a regimen of daily injections for a subsequent seven months to cure lingering cases of osteomyelitis and diskitis in the lumbar region of my spine.

Hooked to the catheter, I felt tethered to my bed–immobile and completely useless. This was both physically and emotionally debilitating for me, not to mention *dehumanizing*. After more than 20 years of an exciting physical career and life, suddenly I was an invalid! Now, of course, I fully believed that I was going to recover, if for no other reason than I simply had the will and the resolve to recover successfully.

And I did–thanks to my personal "cocktail" of Epivir, Zerit and Viramune, with an Amoxycillin chaser to check the re-emergence of the osteomyelitis. It was during this process that I took on the practice of questioning–and at times, countering–the opinions of my various doctors. My numerous years of homeopathy had taught me to be actively involved, and educated about, my own sense of healing–so I wasn't about to relent now! As a matter of fact, it was here where *the Internet* became my friend–providing me with invaluable information on the various medications, their side effects, their combinations, etc. This episode served to place me on a retroviral regimen which I continue to practice to this day. And now, in Winter, 2003, I can look at T-cells in the upper 500s and an undetectable viral load.

Admittedly, I regret that homeopathy wasn't more effective in fighting off the spread of the virus. However, I'm glad that at least I tried it. It was important for me to involve myself in what I felt was a natural and "pro-active" way of trying to heal myself, rather than just relying on manufactured drugs to do the job. Somehow it seemed as if HIV had become a challenge to my system and I had chosen to meet that challenge the best way I knew, even if I did have to finally capitulate to HIV medications to see me out of the darkness.

ANOTHER CHALLENGE

So, imagine my surprise at being diagnosed in August, 2001 with prostate cancer. Now, I believe this developed as the result of a series of testosterone injections I received from my doctor between April and August of that year. Within my "sex-circuit" circle of friends, especially the sexually active gay men, testosterone is widely used. I feel compelled to make my situation as public as possible in order to help other gay men in testosterone-driven circumstances similar to mine; and to call the alarm for them to monitor their PSA levels regularly. By the time my doctor and I checked my PSA level in August–at my *own* request, I might add–it was a whopping 20.5, with a Gleason of 7!

Okay, on to my urologist for an ultrasound, anal probe and biopsy, to discover that I had prostate cancer. I suddenly found myself in the unenviable position of having to surmount yet another obstacle on the road to perfect health. Admittedly, hearing the word "cancer" didn't seem to frighten me; after all, I'd been through the horrors concomitant with HIV, so prostate cancer seemed like a "walk-in-the-park" in comparison.

My previous experience with various doctors around my "HIV saga" had taught me to take considerable time in educating myself about what prostate cancer is, how it develops, and how to treat it. In my humble opinion, had I been this diligent during the months in which I was receiving those lovely testosterone shots in my butt every fortnight, I might have had the wherewithal to "counsel" my doctor to monitor my PSA level more closely. Of course I no longer receive the shots–but how I miss those "baseball biceps."

SURGERY OVER ALTERNATIVE HEALING

My first inclination was to treat it homeopathically with Saw Palmetto, Lycopene, Squalene, etc. However, when my doctor informed me that I should be concerned that the cancer might spread outside the prostate, and the first place it might spread to was my back, I knew it was time for more drastic measures. After all, I had already survived that dreadful summer of 1999–and I was not about to chance having anything happen to my back like that again. I now truly believe in that old adage, "whatever doesn't kill you makes you stronger."

So, as I was now going into my 11th year of sero-conversion, in February, 2002, I elected to have seed implant surgery as my preferred treatment for curing over radiation therapy, hormone therapy or radical prostatectomy, because as a sex club owner and sex-positive and extremely sexually active gay man, I simply couldn't afford to sacrifice either my libido or my erection; they were, and still are, both vitally important to me.

As I was now facing the onslaught of yet another, albeit not as frightening, disease, my original intention to address the situation homeopathically, as I had done after sero-converting to HIV a decade earlier, clearly evaporated.

The Valentine's Day Seed Implant Surgery went especially well, with no problems at all. In fact, I was able to go in at dawn and leave by 4 p.m. that same day unescorted; not, however, until having to throw a veritable "hissy fit" after waiting for more than an hour for a changing shift of nurses, before I had to practically beg one to "dislodge" the Foley Catheter from "my buddy." Here was yet another dehumanizing experience.

A year later I happily find myself *back* to the picture of perfect health! My latest PSA was 4.5, and both libido and erection are in, shall we say, "tip-top shape." Yes, there is still intermittent burning during urination. And I have become almost addicted to Flomax, especially after having missed a series of doses and having landed in the hospital again with a bladder infection that came hairs close to a renal infection. And okay, yes, my ejaculate nowadays is practically non-existent. I have, literally, "dribbles" of cum. Now, that was never really terribly important to me anyway. I always just thought of it as the sort-of "icing on the cake." To me the orgasm itself was always the thing. But I did use to think of it as quite "manly" to watch my eruption of volumes of juice. I have learned to let go of that image of manhood.

Still, the orgasm has returned intact–after a slight detour. Shortly, after my diagnosis, I was introduced, by a dear friend, suffering with the same disease, to a Prostate Cancer Support Group. I lasted barely two meetings. My being openly, outwardly, some might say, even "frighteningly" gay was quite daunting to the predominantly heterosexual men in the room–and, who knows, may have even caused some of the other gay men to look askance. Certainly my open admission to being a sex club owner, and my avid enthusiasm for sexual freedom of expression–being both sex-positive and sexually active–left a somewhat heavy, certainly palpable, discomfort in a room where most men were more concerned about incontinence than about potency or performance.

But then, the *Gay* Prostate Cancer Support Group–*hallelujah!* It was here where I was able to embrace, and more important, discuss this sexual freedom openly, as well as to compare notes on desire, potency, performance, orgasm, and ejaculate; and I stop there, because it was in this group where I discovered the concept of the "missed moment."

I knew it was happening to *me*–that moment while you're masturbating when you're just about to cum, the physical crest of the moment and then it subsides, with nothing coming out. I actually thought it was just me until it came up in the group and several guys chimed in with their own "missed moment" experiences. I guess at that point my old resolve kicked in, and I decided that my next series of masturbatory experiences would *all* end in orgasm–*or else!* Well, I have to admit, there were some nights of close-to, sometimes-more-than, a hour of sweat and strain; but I've now jumped over that hurdle as well, and I'm back to my ol' easygoing masturbating self.

Suffice it to say, this latest struggle to maintain my personal sense of superior health and well-being has most certainly left me with a few "life lessons." First of all, I've had to become aware of the importance of my identity as an African American gay man, a man of color, in continuing to maintain a sense of personal good health.

My several visits to both my oncologist and my urologist consistently placed me in the company of other "mature" African American and Latino men, also in their waiting rooms, which eventually made me think, "Wow, I guess prostate cancer really does seem to adversely affect older men of color. Doesn't that mean that as older men of color we have perhaps an even more serious responsibility to pay diligent attention to our own health, if we're *so* seemingly susceptible to this disease?"

And the answer is, yes, that is exactly what that means! As men of color we don't have the luxury of assuming that the society in which we live is going to look out for our best interests. We really can't take anything for granted–certainly not our "assumed" civil and human rights, and, in this case, not even our dependence on a society that will assist us in watching out for our own physical health. We really have to become much more proactive in keeping ourselves physically healthy–constantly, and vigilantly, watching our health and maintaining our *own* sense of physical security and independence.

This was somewhat of an epiphany for me–because I may have taken such reliance on physical well-being as a given when I was younger, but I don't anymore. I know now, even more than ever, that I'm not a passive, but an extremely active, partner in maintaining my own sense of well-being.

Second, my experience with my various doctors has further underscored similar revelations I've had in the now, more than 12 years of dealing with HIV, that our doctors, unfortunately, simply don't know everything. In many instances, they know barely more than those of us who consistently take the time to search the Internet and process with our friends and support group partners in similar circumstances about how to navigate the vicissitudes of having and enduring HIV and AIDS.

In their defense, it's not all their fault. They've got caseloads of patients; they're basically hitting-the-ground-running. They're doing their best trying to keep their patients healthy. They simply don't have the time to do the research or the processing that so many of us patients do to find out what's wrong with us, and how we can rectify those wrongs.

Nevertheless, I still think it is important whenever necessary to hold our doctors' "feet-to-the-fire" and to challenge their decisions about our possible health solutions when we don't feel they accurately reflect our particular demographic or individual characteristics. I consistently have to remind all my doctors that I'm a gay man and that means a veritable host of different circumstances with which to contend; everything from diet, to sexual practices, to pill-taking regimens and discipline, to, at times, specific drug and substance abuse choices.

Case in point: Upon leaving the clinic after my seed-implant surgery, I was informed by the attending nurse about the various circumstances in which I had to be careful, since I now had radioactive iodine seeds in my prostate, and perhaps my semen as well, i.e., don't impregnate women, refrain from having children sit in my lap, things like that.

Well, dear reader, by this point you must have a sense of me. I instantly countered with, "That's not at all applicable to me! What about masturbation? Am I going to have to throw away a towel immediately afterward because it has radioactive ejaculate? Just how lethal is the little cum he may have from a guy who's been seeded? Is oral and anal sex safe for or to anyone after seeding? What about all those questions?"

She replied, after closing her dropped jaw, "Well, we don't have any data on that." To which I immediately replied, somewhat smugly, I admit, "Well, you should consider to whom you're speaking. I'm a gay man; I have a completely different set of circumstances here, so unless you can address those, you're not really talking to me, are you?"

Now of course, I realize that everyone can't be as "frighteningly-out" as I am. But I still contend that it is about making our doctors as educated as possible. They need our specific, distinctly different information. And my feeling is that if you come across a doctor who seems to "cookie-cutter" you into a category recognizable to him, and thereby prescribe a solution, a remedy, or a choice of operation to you having absolutely no awareness of your specific, individual needs as a gay man–well, keep going 'til you find a doctor who will listen. Because after all, we really do have different sets of circumstances with which we have to contend and we deserve to be treated accordingly.

Living with Prostate Cancer:
One Gay Man's Experience

Jerry Harris

SUMMARY. The author, a gay man diagnosed with prostate cancer at age 48, describes his experience deciding on a course of treatment and coping with sexual dysfunction following a prostatectomy. His experience was made more difficult by ignorance in the medical community, the straight community and the gay community. Frustrated by the absence of a source of fully accepting and understanding support, he started his own support group for gay men with prostate cancer. *[Article copies available for a fee from The Haworth Document Delivery Service: 1-800-HAWORTH. E-mail address: <docdelivery@haworthpress.com> Website: <http://www.HaworthPress.com> © 2005 by The Haworth Press, Inc. All rights reserved.]*

KEYWORDS. Dry orgasm, erectile dysfunction, gay community, gay support group, prostate cancer, prostatectomy, sexual dysfunction, support group

I received the diagnosis of prostate cancer the weekend of my 48th birthday (1996). The previous month a routine PSA blood test produced

---

Jerry Harris holds a PhD in sociology from the University of Oregon. He is a computer programmer for a financial corporation.

[Haworth co-indexing entry note]: "Living with Prostate Cancer: One Gay Man's Experience." Harris, Jerry. Co-published simultaneously in *Journal of Gay & Lesbian Psychotherapy* (The Haworth Medical Press, an imprint of The Haworth Press, Inc.) Vol. 9, No. 1/2, 2005, pp. 109-117; and: *A Gay Man's Guide to Prostate Cancer* (ed: Gerald Perlman, and Jack Drescher) The Haworth Medical Press, an imprint of The Haworth Press, Inc., 2005, pp. 109-117. Single or multiple copies of this article are available for a fee from The Haworth Document Delivery Service [1-800-HAWORTH, 9:00 a.m. - 5:00 p.m. (EST). E-mail address: docdelivery@haworthpress.com].

a 4.8 score, barely above the 4.0 considered normal. Given that the digital exam didn't suggest a problem and I didn't have any symptoms, neither my primary care doctor nor my urologist had been particularly concerned. Following a second PSA score of 5.1, the urologist performed a biopsy. The positive result was shocking. Given the nature of all the results, he was quite sure the cancer was limited within the prostate gland itself. With that diagnosis and my age, he strongly recommended a prostatectomy (removal of the prostate) as a way to ensure total elimination of the cancer.

WHAT THE DOCTOR'S OFFICE DOESN'T TELL YOU

By that point I had done a little research; I knew there was risk to my sexual functioning. I had acquired a videotape of a recently aired Public Broadcasting Station special on prostate cancer, on which my urologist had been interviewed. Not surprisingly, none of the patients interviewed were gay-identified. Next to the issue of which treatment option would most effectively eliminate my cancer, my primary concern was the effect of treatment on sexual functioning. So when the urologist offered to connect me with other patients who had had the operation, I told him I was gay and would appreciate contact with gay patients.

My doctor's nurse contacted one of his patients whom they knew was gay; he had had the surgery six months earlier. That evening, the man (I'll name him Tom) called me. In the next few weeks, I spoke with him several times, sharing intimate information strangers rarely do. He thankfully never hesitated to respond to my questions. The first thing Tom asked was if I knew about "dry orgasms." I didn't. I learned from him that, after a prostatectomy, a man can still feel an orgasm but cannot ejaculate. I felt more stunned by this than by the diagnosis. And I felt ashamed at my ignorance; I should have known what the prostate does and that this therefore would be a consequence of removing it. I have realized since that, despite my many years of higher education, I am part of a large population of men ignorant about how our bodies function.

And later, looking back on that moment, I felt angry; because even then I was one step ahead of where Tom had been before *his* operation. He hadn't learned about loss of ejaculation until he was in his hospital room, recovering from the operation, reading a book about prostate cancer! No doctor–not our urologist, and none of those either of us consulted for second and third opinions–ever brought this up!

Although their silence may simply reflect their assumptions about what patients know, I wonder if it also reflects heterosexual ignorance of gay males' sexual lives. Not ejaculating has different implications for gay men. Most heterosexual men's primary sexual activity is intercourse. Since most prostate cancer patients are over fifty and probably not concerned with child-bearing, not ejaculating has little consequence for straight men. A man ejaculates inside the woman. If he has a dry orgasm (feeling an orgasm but not producing fluid), absence of fluid is irrelevant to sexual satisfaction. For many gay men, however, watching our partners and/or ourselves having an orgasm is an integral part of our sexual experience, especially in this age of safer sex. Not preparing gay patients (and all patients) for this consequence of prostate cancer treatment is a gross disservice.

Tom assured me that after the prostatectomy I would still feel the sensation of an orgasm, which indeed is the case. However, erectile functioning is a different issue, varying from patient to patient. My personal decision was to delay confronting this issue until after my operation. Partly this was based on hopeful statistics indicating that younger prostatectomy patients are more likely to regain erectile functioning; but for me sexual functioning took a back seat to finding the best way to get rid of the cancer.

Also tucked away until later was the experience Tom related to me with a boyfriend of six months. His boyfriend provided support during his recovery from the operation, but several months later ended the relationship. He said Tom's inability to have erections, a condition Tom still hoped would improve, was not why he broke it off; Tom believed otherwise. I wondered with some trepidation if such issues were to be in my future too.

LACK OF SUPPORT–STRAIGHT OR GAY

About six weeks after diagnosis, I had a prostatectomy. While all indications were that my operation was a success (six years later, I still show no signs of cancer!), I was not one of the lucky ones as far as erectile functioning is concerned. Two months after the operation, I started attending support meetings of *Us Too*, a national organization of support groups for men with prostate cancer. I found the meetings to be gay-tolerant, but not gay-friendly; this reflected as much the behavior of the participants as the group leaders. In phone conversations, I informed several organizers I was gay and was assured I was welcome. My optimism waned during the meetings. The few times I spoke up in the groups regarding sexual activity, any responses assumed heterosexual behavior. And when I prefaced my comments by saying I was gay, either no one responded or responses were from their heterosexual experiences. While I didn't feel hostility, I did experience a sense of aloneness. If there were gay men there, and I eventually learned there were, they weren't acknowledging themselves.

Since coming out in my early twenties, whenever I needed support, I sought out gay organizations. However, compounding my difficulties in confronting my erectile dysfunction issues was the absence of any support within the gay community. Having volunteered in various gay counseling organizations throughout life, I was disappointed to find an absence of knowledgeable support (other than good luck wishes) from gay health clinics, AIDS organizations, gay counseling centers, a gay switchboard and an organization for gay seniors. The New York City office for lesbian and gay health issues had no referrals to offer me. The isolation I had experienced at *Us Too* seemed less pronounced than what I felt during my search among gay groups: This was *my* community failing me. Did one need to have AIDS or a sexually transmitted disease before we responded to each other's needs?

ISSUES I NEEDED TO DISCUSS

Five months post-operative, I went to my surgeon's colleague, a sexual dysfunction specialist. Initially I delayed seeing him, hoping I might naturally regain my erectile functioning, but men in *Us Too* urged me not to wait. Ideally, I should have been told earlier that frequent sexual stimulation and using any artificial or medicinal aids as soon as possible after the operation improves the chances of stimulating erectile activity. At the time, Viagra (sildenafil) did not exist. (Unfortunately, it is ineffective for a significant proportion of men who have had a prostatectomy. It doesn't work for me.) Other available options, each with its drawbacks, include vacuum devices, penile injections, the "MUSE" (an intraurethral pellet) or a penile implant. How one assesses the benefits and drawbacks of each is largely subjective. Having gay men to discuss these options with would have been invaluable in those early months. It felt very frustrating sorting out the options on my own.

I also had all sorts of questions about sexual and social situations: Are there ways of getting through a sexual encounter without a partner knowing I can't get hard? Is cruising a guy on a nude beach or in a steam room no longer possible? When I meet a guy I'm interested in, when do I tell him about my problem: before a date, before we go home, before we get into bed or not at all? The decision–if and when to share the "secret"–seems similar in some respects to the dilemma facing an HIV-positive man. When, if at all, do I speak up? I discussed these questions with a couple of friends, who listened sympathetically but didn't know how to respond. I wanted something like an AIDS-support group, but for gay men with prostate cancer. There was none to be found. I questioned myself: was I exaggerating the importance of these questions? No. The feelings of isolation, frustration and anger I felt became clarified during a brief vacation. I met a man in a bar, a rare experience for me. On our way back to my hotel, I told him of my problem having erections. He seemed okay with it, but after a few kisses he lay down on his stomach. Did he want a massage? To be slapped? Was he turned off? He must have understood from what I had said that I couldn't penetrate him. Shortly later he left. I never expected much from a bar pickup, but I knew I needed other men with whom to sort out the self-doubts that the incident touched.

FINDING SUPPORT–AND IGNORANCE

During the next half year, I made an effort to start a monthly support group for gay men with prostate cancer. Living in New York City, it was relatively easy to develop a list of doctors, therapists and counselors with large gay clientele. I distributed a flyer to them as well as to the gay organizations I had sought support from earlier in the year. *Us Too* let me put the flyer on the information table at its meetings; most of my respondents came from those (apparently heterosexual) meetings. I created a web page. (Web responses were few. At that time internet users were primarily younger people and prostate cancer is diagnosed primarily in older men.) There were enough responses so that a year after my operation, a monthly group started meeting in my home. The first night reminded me of my feeling when attending my first coming out group 25 years earlier–the exhilarating feeling of finally finding others who understood how I felt, with whom I could talk without having to explain or justify each thought and reaction.

The group lasted for three years. It included numerous men who came only once or twice and a few regulars who attended for at least a year. Participants ranged from my age to a man in his eighties. Issues discussed included explicitly sexual situations, social situations and medical issues. For two of the men incontinence was an issue, a problem I fortunately never faced except for a few post-operative weeks. One of the older men talked about how the vacuum pump became a new toy when having sex with his long-time lover. One man discussed complications that arose after having a penile implant. (He required two corrective operations.) Discussion ranged from being instructive to being scary to being humorous.

In the three years the group met, none of the men I talked with were able to be the active partner in penile-rectal intercourse. I'm ignorant about heterosexual intercourse, but my impression is that penile-rectal sex requires a firmer erection than penile-vaginal sex. I believe that the stated effectiveness of the available options for erectile dysfunction exclude the realities of penile-rectal penetration; and hence much of the gay male sexual experience. I also wonder if studies of the proportion of men who achieve "satisfactory" erectile functioning after prostate cancer treatment include a representative number of gay men–and if statistical breakouts between heterosexual and homosexual respondents would show different results.

The group was a welcome contrast to the *Us Too* group's assumption that all men's sexuality is the same. That same assumption also pervaded the books and articles I had found. The widely recommended book, *The Prostate: A Guide for Men and the Women Who Love Them* (1995) said it all in its title. I had to "translate" heterosexual sexual references into my own experience. Indeed, if my hypothesis is correct–if what is a "satisfactory" erection varies for gay and straight sexual experiences–then gay men may not be "translating" correctly, and thus may be making decisions about choice of treatment based on misinformation.

One couple attended several group sessions. The younger man, there to support his partner who had undergone radiation therapy, talked about how participants in an *Us Too* partner's support group initially were resistant to his participation, since only wives had previously been in the group. His partner talked about having to urinate in the bushes outside his building on the way home from a radiation treatment. (Such treatments can cause temporary incontinence.) A policeman arrested him and it required a court appearance, before a thankfully understanding judge, to dismiss the charge. Both incidents had an impact on the rest of the group. They made me angry. Even when confronting prostate cancer, gay men had to be ready to cope with homophobia and stupidity.

And I was both angered and saddened, but not surprised, to find such ignorance within the gay community. Sexual dysfunction, illness and aging are issues gay men prefer to avoid. The possibility of prostate cancer raises all these fears. One of the group members and I set up an information table at the New York City Lesbian and Gay Community Center's annual garden party. We counted fewer than thirty people who approached our table in three hours, out of over a thousand attendees; and at least half of them had primarily a professional interest (counselors, ministers, nurses). This was reminiscent of reactions I had in the 1980s, trying to leaflet men in gay bars about safe sex.

Shortly after Viagra came on the market, but before it became used as a recreational drug, I was in a chat room where someone was booted out for mentioning it. Another participant remarked, "We don't need Viagra in this chat room." This short exchange made me feel like a pariah.

Of course, any gay man who has spent time in chat rooms looking to meet other gay men knows that, while one can get into enjoyable discussions and even meet someone, there is a fair amount of vacuous give and take as well. I had to endure exchanges which, following my prostatectomy, intermittently wounded or angered me at least momentarily, despite my knowing they weren't worthy of serious concern. I always rejected the idea of being a "top" or "bottom" in or out of bed, but my sexual limitations made me sensitive to being asked which I was. More graphically, being asked how big my erection was, or if I "shoot a big load," was something I couldn't shrug off quite as easily as I could before the operation.

My generally optimistic attitude was challenged by such ignorance. Fortunately, a year and a half after the operation, I had an experience that boosted my morale. I met a man at my gym who was visiting the city. During the course of the summer, we spent several erotic, obviously mutually satisfying afternoons together. Unlike earlier encounters I had had since the operation, he was as focused on my pleasure as on his own. He seemed to enjoy oral sex even though I was never more than semi-erect. And he enthusiastically engaged in prolonged mutual masturbation, a variety of penetration "techniques" not involving an erection, as well as the pleasures of kissing, embracing and massage. By summer's end, I was encouraged that indeed a healthy attitude about sex was more important than one's physical limitations; I still could believe that there was a man "out there" for me somewhere.

Still, not wanting to leave any stone unturned, after the summer I tried penile injections as a means to get an erection. The MUSE (an intraurethral pellet) had only been partially effective; and my urologist said the injections were the most effective alternative. The thought of self-injection had discouraged me until then. One patient in my doctor's office had praise for the injections, assuring me self-injection was a breeze, but it took all the emotional strength I could muster to attempt it. While the nurses in the office instructed me well, it took several efforts at home before finally injecting myself. The medicine worked too well. My erection never subsided; after three hours, I had to go to the emergency room and be treated with an antidote. My doctor reduced my dosage to one-third the original amount, but I was never again able to work through my mental block to inject myself. An injection as part of foreplay just wouldn't do for me. And my summer experience was encouragement enough for me to decide that I could have a sex life with my sexual functioning as it is.

SIGNS OF CHANGE

I equate my effort to start the support group to a graduate school experience in the 1970s, when I initiated an experimental sociology course on my campus on the gay experience. In attempting to fill a personal support need (in the 1970s, coming out; now, living with prostate cancer), I had to become an activist. A listing for our prostate cancer group in several local gay publications attracted several writers. One interviewer included my story in a book published on gay health issues. And the *Dallas Voice*, learning of our group from the web page, interviewed me for a feature on prostate cancer in the gay community. To publicize the support group, I arranged for a panel of members of our group to speak to SAGE (Senior Action in a Gay Environment). The panel attracted mostly men in their 60s and older. During the second year of our group, we looked for a more permanent location. We found a "home" in New York's Callen-Lorde Community Health Center, which provided a free meeting space and gave us a listing in their newsletter.

While these bits of "celebrity" were uplifting, they had stemmed from a very personal need. I would have much preferred if the support mechanisms I required had existed when I most needed them. Having a full-time job, I found maintaining publicity for the group burdensome. (Attendance waned during its third year. I eventually discontinued it.) Fortunately, in the past two years, there finally are appearing bits of supportive activity within the gay community for men with prostate cancer. About three years ago, a web chat network was started for gay men with prostate cancer or having other prostate issues; it can be reached at *prostate-owner@groups.queernet.org*. In the spring of 2002 St. Vincent's Hospital in New York started a group similar to the one I had started.

And in October, someone in the chat network sent out a notice that the University of California in San Francisco had started a similar group.

Personally, attending the St. Vincent's group was more rewarding than my own. I could focus more on my own needs and less on the group dynamics. A lot of the questions I had several years ago have been answered by the opportunities I have had to talk with other men and by working through personal experiences; but I still feel the occasional need to share this aspect of who I am with others. Unfortunately, not every prostate cancer patient lives happily ever after. Even as the likelihood of it re-emerging becomes more remote with each passing annual PSA check-up, I can never fully divorce myself from that possibility. And there will probably always be moments when I wish my body functioned better sexually. As I write this, I am looking forward to a Saturday night date with a man whom I met eight months ago, my first relationship since many years preceding my diagnosis. To my surprise, my sexual limitations seem largely irrelevant to the intimacy we enjoy. I think my emotional struggle to cope with prostate cancer has been more important to our relationship; it helps me take less for granted and cherish more what I can have.

REFERENCE

Walsh, P.C. & Worthington, J.F. (1995), *The Prostate: A Guide for Men and the Women Who Love Them*. Baltimore: The Johns Hopkins University Press.

Identity and Prostate Cancer: Comments on a Messy Life

"Mark Miller"

SUMMARY. The author's image of his body as small and weak was formed as a child but has remained with him although he is no longer physically weak. At times of emotional stress, he is susceptible to poor body image. A radical prostatectomy done after being diagnosed with prostate cancer eliminated the reliability of the author's erections and gravely affected his identity. In his recovery from surgery, the author realized that having reliable erections, not as a condition to sexual pleasure but simply having them, was a part of his identity. In the aftermath of cancer and major surgery, he doubts that his body will appear appealing to other gay men. In light of the after-effects of radical prostatectomy, and in consideration of intimations of mortality, he worries that he will not be loved. *[Article copies available for a fee from The Haworth Document Delivery Service: 1-800-HAWORTH. E-mail address: <docdelivery@haworthpress. com> Website: <http://www.HaworthPress.com> © 2005 by The Haworth Press, Inc. All rights reserved.]*

KEYWORDS. Body image, coming out, depression, erections, external identity, gay men, identity, internal identity, prostate cancer, prostatectomy

The author is a professional living in New York City. He was diagnosed with prostate cancer at age 52.

Some names (including the author's) and identifying details have been altered.

[Haworth co-indexing entry note]: "Identity and Prostate Cancer: Comments on a Messy Life." "Miller, Mark." Co-published simultaneously in *Journal of Gay & Lesbian Psychotherapy* (The Haworth Medical Press, an imprint of The Haworth Press, Inc.) Vol. 9, No. 1/2, 2005, pp. 119-129; and: *A Gay Man's Guide to Prostate Cancer* (ed: Gerald Perlman, and Jack Drescher) The Haworth Medical Press, an imprint of The Haworth Press, Inc., 2005, pp. 119-129. Single or multiple copies of this article are available for a fee from The Haworth Document Delivery Service [1-800-HAWORTH, 9:00 a.m. - 5:00 p.m. (EST). E-mail address: docdelivery@haworthpress.com].

http://www.haworthpress.com/web/JGLP
© 2005 by The Haworth Press, Inc. All rights reserved.
Digital Object Identifier: 10.1300/J236v09n01_10

"Being gay is about 15% of who I am." That's what I said when the facilitator of our gay men's prostate cancer support group asked us to describe our experiences of prostate cancer "as gay men." My identity includes abilities, disabilities, values and interests. Some of these relate to being gay. Most do not.

I underwent a radial prostatectomy at age 53, about a year before writing this account. Prostate cancer has surprised me in that it has shown me parts of my identity I did not realize were there, or whose importance I did not appreciate. The prostate is not one of God's better creations. The conception is fine; the execution is lousy. It is in the middle of everything anatomically, and, it turns out, it is right in the middle of everything about being a man.

While I am without doubt exclusively homosexual in orientation and sexual history, I hardly feel qualified to comment about anything "as a gay man." What follows derives exclusively from my own feelings and experience (except where a specific reference is indicated). If readers find some truth of general applicability therein, so much the better, but that is not my intention.

My coming-out has been the longest, slowest and most incomplete in history. It would be more accurate to say, "my comings-out," because, as I allude to above, being gay is not the only way I identify myself to myself. There are comings-out more difficult than the gay one, even in New York, the second gayest city in America. Being alone, feeling lonely, having depression, bipolar disorder, type II, to be exact, are some other important comings-out I have had to negotiate.

I have been depressed as long as I can remember, at least since age 12. It was only diagnosed as bipolar, as opposed to unipolar depression, when I was in my forties. The typical course is a general low-level depression, with major depressive episodes that can last a few months occurring every three or four years, and occasional hypomanic episodes of no more than a day, which come about 3 times a year, usually right after a major depressive episode. As it happens, this past year, I started having hypomanic episodes 3 or 4 times a day; but we adjusted my meds, and that stopped. Since the prostatectomy, however, I have been in a rather major depressive state almost all the time, going on a year now. I have never been hospitalized for depression, and I cannot imagine why. I manage to keep myself clothed, fed and employed, which is likewise a mystery to me.

I am just old enough to remember that the phrase "coming-out" used to have a different meaning. It used to mean coming out to yourself, that is, realizing you were gay. In those pre-Stonewall days, it was assumed that this was a process, because being gay was simply not an option, and realizing that you were gay involved a lot of work. Now, however, that meaning is forgotten, and the phrase means not only acknowledging that identity to oneself, but declaring it to others as well. This difference between an internal identity (how you recognize yourself) and an external identity (how you are seen) is an important distinction for me.

A complicated identity may be a source of strength to others, but for me, it is just messy. I do not feel that I fit anywhere and I do want to fit somewhere. Prostate cancer has further muddled and weakened elements of this messy identity, and increased my isolation. I find myself far from the center; an eccentric, damaged, bipolar individual who talks too much. However, I am not rich enough, smart enough or handsome enough to get away with being eccentric, so it means a lot of covering up, and it is tiring.

For me, a specifically gay issue of having prostate cancer is an exaggerated importance of physical attractiveness. Body image is a major factor for me, and since cancer has hit me in all my weakest points, that has been a crucial one for my identities: how I see myself, and how I am seen.

IDENTITIES

It is sometimes surprising to me which attributes end up as a part of identity. I recall someone at a tenants' meeting beginning a question by saying "I'm a dog-owner." I think I would have just said, "I own a dog;" but clearly her identity as a dog-owner meant a lot more than that to her.

I am equally surprised by which elements have formed my identity. I was born into an assimilated, non-observant Jewish family. My mother's role model is June Cleaver, not Golda Meir. I am a member of no Jewish organization, never go to synagogue, and even, according to strictest Jewish law, do not have a Jewish name, so that I could not participate in any formal way in Jewish life. Yet my Jewish identity is my strongest identity, because I feel connected, not horizontally to other Jews now living, but vertically to all my forebears and to all Jews in past generations. It is, however, being connected to *a* people, rather than to people, which is an abstraction, not a feeling.

I am passionately interested in opera and have learned quite a bit about it over the years. I know operaphiles who go to the opera twenty times more often than I do and know a hundred times more than I do, yet

I think of myself as an operaphile, and not merely someone who goes to the opera a dozen times a year.

On the other hand, what I do for a living and whom I want to sleep with are only secondary ways in which I recognize myself. They take up a lot of time, energy and sometimes pain and heartbreak. They govern where and how I spend much of my time, but they are not much of who I am.

I have reluctantly come to the conclusion that we live in a virtual state I call Gay Nation. This is a state whose founding principles are liberty, the pursuit of happiness, but above all, looking good. Looking good includes a good haircut and fashionable clothes, but most of all, having the right body. Gay Nation is not a republic and not exactly a monarchy, but it is a kind of meritocracy. The merit is how good you look. The constitution of Gay Nation, and especially of its elite, is well described in Daniel Mendelsohn's (1999) brilliant *Elusive Embrace*.

We are not all good citizens of Gay Nation. I certainly am not. I do not observe the secular high holy days of Oscar Night and Halloween. I do not engage in the preferred entertainments of dance clubs, party drugs, going into debt for Prada and indiscriminate tricking. I never got the point of Cher, fabulousness or drag. Most important, I do not look right. A friend who grew up red-haired in the Middle East says she knows what it is to be "the wrong kind of person" because of how you look. I am definitely the wrong kind of person in Gay Nation.

We may reject the values of Gay Nation; we may not observe its laws; we may break them; but it takes a very strong or very lucky man to ignore them. In one way or another, it is the standard against which we (except for the strong or lucky few) measure ourselves, whether we acknowledge it or not. This is where we live.

I am short and thin, wear glasses, and look, in brief, like a geek. Other gay men may see lean, but they do not see sexy. My handsome friend Dan stopped by New York for a few days on his way to visit his parents about a month after my prostate surgery. Dan was wonderful: carried groceries, hooked up my new phone, gave hugs, encouraged me to go out with him, but gave me room to be alone. One day when I was complaining about my life, he said, "You have a great life! You have a terrific apartment, you have good job, you travel the world, you speak six languages, you have so many interests. . . ." "None of which will get me laid," I said. Dan said nothing. He knew I was right.

Nora Ephron (1975) wrote that she would have been a different person if she had had bigger breasts. She would have been. Men would have looked at her differently, or, simply, they would have looked at her. Ephron is a brilliant comic writer. She might have written the following scene, set in a gay bar. Two friends are standing at one end, and one says to the other "You see that guy over there with the glasses and the bad haircut? Someone told me he can calculate square roots in his head and he volunteers at a homeless shelter three nights a week." His friend says, "Man, that is so hot! Do you think I'd have a chance with him?" In a movie, this would be hilarious. In real life, the converse is not. In Gay Nation, even if I am seen, I am not valued; in particular, my sexual nature (including the fact that I have a sexual nature) is invisible.

Before prostate cancer, I had been aware that erection, ejaculation, and orgasm were three separate phenomena, governed by three different neural pathways. I knew that after prostatectomy, there would be no ejaculation, and thought that it would not matter to me. I was wrong. Because all three had always occurred together, it was impossible to imagine what each might be like independently. It has been odd, and not satisfying.

For some reason, perhaps my geeky appearance, no one suspected that I had a large erection. (Perhaps I still have it.) I did not even realize it until I had been around the block quite a few times. It comes as a surprise in intimate situations. I had never had occasion to appreciate what having reliable erections meant to me until prostate cancer ravaged it. Wholly apart from being a condition to sexual pleasure, it is, it seems, a part of my identity. It was just something I had, and until I no longer had it, I never realized that it was a part of who I am. Without reliable erections, I do not feel like myself.

The size of my erection has nothing to do with the degree of pleasure I could give or experience. The size of my erection never meant much to me, but it seems to have meant a lot to others. If it meant a lot to others, well then, I guess, in fact, that means something to me. It is also, more or less, a secret, and it is a secret I liked having.

Here is an interesting paradox, at the intersection of the internal and external identities. In Gay Nation, it is the external, the large erection, that counts, not the sexual sensitivity I might have had.

BODY IMAGE AND BODILY REALITY

Physically weak and always the smallest in my class, as I was throughout childhood and school years, I was not at ease in my body. There was no growth spurt in adolescence. Puberty started early but drifted along slowly. I was still growing in college. It was not like a certain junior high school classmate, who in June of seventh grade was a pretty ephebe with a high voice and the next September was a colt with pecs and hair. Of the many humiliations, I can recall from that year was an unsuccessful attempt to run hurdles. The gym teacher singled me out and called me a girl.

My image of my body was accurate then: small and weak. My physical weakness as a child and as a young person caused me to worry constantly about my physical security. Even though I only got beaten up once, my little body made me feel vulnerable all the time. It never occurred to me that strength of intellect could be protective as well.

I had no confidence that I could ever become strong, but somehow I tricked myself into running, and then later going to a gym, both just before I turned 30. Eventually I got to be good at running and did, in fact, become rather strong. Even on my worst days, I could run three or four miles. I came to realize that this meant I could count on being able to get myself three miles away from anything, with nothing but my legs. Running did, however, come to an end after a serious knee injury sustained in an automobile accident a few years after I started running. I did not become big and muscular, but I could bench press 150% of my body weight. I acquired the function of strength but not the appearance of strength. The body changed but the image did not. Knowing (1) I could bench press 150% of my body weight, an objective fact even if it did not show; (2) that other, secret, physical attribute which could also be gauged objectively; and (3) with a whole lot of persuading myself that (1) and (2) were both true and significant, I could on occasion think of myself as a man, without exploding in laughter or tears. Those occasions were rare.

Even after turning from scrawny runt to wiry runt, the persona did not work very well in Gay Nation. When a man, any man, looks at another man's body, he sees pecs, biceps, maybe legs–power and strength, or their absence. This is not how women see men. Gay men see the same power and strength elements, and they also see the things women see: abs, butt, perhaps eyes and hands. For gay men the conventional signifiers of masculinity carry a sexualized meaning, but gay men are men, so these signs still embody strength and power, which are inestimably valued in Gay Nation. In any case, appearance is, as I said, the key. It is the résumé. It may not get you the job but it will decide whether you get the interview.

SCARS

I said that cancer has hit at all my most weak points, and my body image is clearly the weakest. Compounding this was the objective fact that I lost a great deal of weight and strength following surgery. Because of the loss of strength in the months after surgery, I did not just feel that I had the insignificant body I had when I was young, but I actually had it again. Thus began the first post-op depression. I looked like crap, so had no confidence that I would be accepted or even seen in Gay Nation (and did not have much confidence to begin with). No confidence, so no attempts at a connection. Any connection, not merely hooking up, seemed impossible. Someone to talk to would be nice. Someone to kiss and cuddle with would be nicer. No attempts, no successes. No successes, so I really must look like crap. This is faulty logic, but the confidence-skill feedback loop does not run on logic. Shortly after I was diagnosed, I started going to an "all levels" yoga class. When I expressed my frustration to the instructor about how much worse I was than nearly everyone else in the class, he said, "You get good at what you do." The converse is also true: you do not get good at what you do not do. My problem is that without some minimal level of confidence in myself, I cannot put myself into situations where rejection is almost assured. Confidence in myself means confidence in the way I look.

There is now an external scar on my belly, about three inches long. It is not so bad, with one exception. In fact, I wanted a scar as a sign of what I was going to go through. The exception is an odd dimple that looks like a second navel. I am told by several men that it is not that apparent, but it is apparent to me. My dermatologist says that it is barely visible which is a good thing, because he also says there is nothing to do about it. I have, in middle age, a relatively flat belly. Luck and genetics, to be sure, but also a lot of work. Abs are important to the men of Gay Nation. This deformity spoils it.

There are internal scars, in a literal and figurative sense. The literal ones are something I learned about recently, and explain why I am not regaining function as soon as I expected to. I may never regain function fully, and at the moment, things are getting worse. I should not have been surprised: my knee never really healed, and my depression is pretty much untreatable. Lots of messes, everywhere I look.

Thus began the second post-op depression, which continues to this day. I now know that prostate cancer has left scars that will not heal. Confidence in reliable erections is gone. I have not yet devised a strategy for dealing with this, except, possibly, talking too much, which is counterproductive. And moot. If there were no attempts at connection during the first post-op depression, there surely are none now. This results not merely from the literal loss of function but the damage to identity. I do not feel like myself; I do not feel like anyone. I seemed invisible to others before. Now I feel invisible to myself. After the surgery, I felt like damaged goods; now I know that I am. The security in being able to run three miles away from anything is gone, the 150% bench press is gone, the prostate is gone, the reliable erections are gone.

FLUIDS

It may seem ironic that one of the few places I do not feel bad about my body is on a "nude beach." Horrible locution. In Germany it is called "free-body-culture" and in France and Spain, "naturist." I much prefer these terms because it is there where I feel free and there where I feel a part of nature, and perhaps only there. It is there that I am most comfortable in my body and also the least aware of it. Naturism is not more and not less sexual than everyday life. If I see a beautiful shirtless 22 year-old in a park in the middle of the city, is that not sexual? I might have a caught a break here. Major incontinence would have put an end to naturism, and perhaps thus to the one place where I feel I am a part of the world. I am losing a little ground here recently, but there are exercises that might help.

I also knew that after prostatectomy there would be no semen. I did not think this would be a problem. It was messy anyway. It *has* turned out to be a problem, and I am not sure why. I had no particular attachment to it. I did not view it a sign of masculinity. Perhaps it is just one more signifier of what I have lost.

SOME THOUGHTS ABOUT HOW THE STRAIGHT DOCS TREATED ME

All my doctors are handsome, sexy guys. This has been encouraging, for some reason. They are all straight, but I did not really think they would, in this day and age, fail to value a gay man's orgasm. They explained all the possible side-effects of treatment except one, and described all the potential sexual side-effects. I definitely feared that they might not value a currently unpartnered gay man's orgasm, or assume that a gay man is either "top" or "bottom" and that we all engage in anal sex. However, they never asked about a partner or about particular sexual practices, so neither issue arose. When I now mention that I do not have a regular partner, they do not judge.

The one side-effect they should have told me about is post-operative depression. I gave them all my medical history, and they understood it, and told me which medications to discontinue before anesthesia. They made sure to tell me that I could see a psychiatrist while in the hospital if I wanted. It is really difficult to figure out that you are in a post-operative depression, when you have never heard the term, and did not know it was a possibility. Even really good doctors have misconceptions about mental illness. Did they think that if they mentioned it, it would become a self-fulfilling prophecy? They could tell from talking to me that I am a smart guy and know the ins and outs of depression. They really should have told me. It probably would not have helped with the post-op depression I am in now, but it would have helped with the first one.

The other thing the doctors should have told me was something I heard only from one erectile dysfunction specialist, about how to take Viagra (sildenafil). (By the time this is published, Cialis (tadalafil) may have supplanted Viagra, but this doctor has told me that the same caution applies to Cialis.) This doctor, but no one else, said that during the first 60-90 minutes after taking the drug there should be no sexual simulation whatsoever. "Read The Wall Street Journal," he says. As I understand the biochemistry of erection, it starts when nitric oxide is released in the penis as a neurotransmitter, as a result of sexual stimulation. The process is further mediated by phosphodiesterase-5 (PDE-5), one of many enzymes involved in erection. This specialist's advice made sense, and he later confirmed to me that until the PDE-5 is completely blocked, any nitric oxide produced by stimulation is wasted, and after 90 minutes, you are going to run out of nitric oxide. Not even Pfizer tells you this, let alone any of the other urologists I have consulted. This information, it seems, must be passed from hand to hand, samizdat-style, and I am doing my part.

THE ODDS

What are the odds? My mother taught us early on that although we were assimilated and non-observant Jews, we were Jews first of all, but this identity was to be concealed, if at all possible. There are a lot of mixed messages in there, and especially a lot for a child to handle. She also made it very clear that it was preferable not to have feelings at all, but imperative not to express them. My mother still scolds me for "talking with my hands" or laughing out loud at a play or movie.

If it is shameful to laugh at a comedy, what kind of coming-out, or comings-out, could I have had? And what conversations about sex or death? I am not so much afraid that I will die, but afraid of not knowing what the odds are. No one can tell me. I am trying to figure this out on my own. I am reading medical journals and looking for statistics. I try not to let my mother know any of this because it makes her angry. *Yes, angry. She is angry with me for being scared.* In the past few years, my father, mother, brother, an uncle and several cousins have all had cancer, and they have gone back to work, are playing tennis and sleep at night. They are all better at having cancer than I am. I am breaking the rules.

Needless to say, if I am neither seen nor accepted, the chances of finding love will be, well, chancy. The universe of special men who could see the merits of a small middle-aged man with average looks, social ineptitude, a lack of enthusiasm for show-tunes, depressive illness and a tendency to talk too much is small. So small that I have never found it. Now we add cancer, the scar, the erectile problems, the absence of fluid. . . .

Twenty years ago, my knee surgeon said I would be running in six months. A year ago, I went to sleep with the capacity for that bench press and erections and woke up three hours later without them. The stalled recovery has now put me outside of my latest little corner of identity: recovering prostatectomy patient. Others are getting better but I am not. My body is not behaving itself as it should. As I began to heal, I felt more a part of the world. As my recovery stalls, or reverses, I am dropping out again.

Pre-op, I had been told that the odds were one in five that I would have capsular penetration, i.e., that the cancer would have spread beyond the prostate gland. I drew the one. Post-op, the odds that I would have normal urinary and erectile function by now were in the very high 90's out of 100. Things looked promising for a while, but are reversing course. Thus, when I read that the odds that I will have a recurrence of cancer in five years are one in eleven, or one in three, what am I to think?

One reads of how close brushes with death change people. They quit their boring jobs, do what they always wanted to do, tell rude people to go fuck themselves, and, by the way, find love in the process. Stewart's (2002) recent best-seller tells just such a story. I, on the other hand, am *schlepping* from day to day, still wanting to belong, to be heard, and have a decent erection. A year after surgery, I have started to get my strength back, but it is often one step forward and two steps back. It is eighth grade gym class, and I am not getting over the hurdles.

REFERENCES

Ephron, N. (1975), "A Few Words About Breasts" in *Crazy Salad: Some Things About Women*. NY: Random House.

Mendelsohn, D. (1999), *The Elusive Embrace: Desire and the Riddle of Identity*. NY. Knopf.

Stewart, J. B. (2002), *Heart of a Soldier: A Story of Love, Heroism, and September 11th*. NY: Simon & Schuster.

Prostate Cancer at Age 84

Bertram Schaffner

SUMMARY. A gay man is first diagnosed with prostate cancer at age 84. The cancer is aggressive and requires treatment. He struggles with the choice of treatment. Surgery is inadvisable because the cancer has already advanced beyond the capsule, and surgery raises the danger of possible metastasis. Preservation of erectile potency is ruled out as a cause of concern, since he is no longer sexually potent. Due to the lack of knowledge and experience (as opposed to present-day advances) radiation, in its form at that time, is ruled out. There was danger of radiation burns to adjacent healthy tissue. Chemotherapy was not recommended to him at that time. Patient settled on hormone therapy, deciding that he could manage the consequences of hormonal castration, even though his doctors never discussed his homosexual lifestyle with him. This oversight seemed less important at the time, because the patient was already impotent. Patient's overriding concern was with the formation of a living situation or home with another man, for the remainder of his life. *[Article copies available for a fee from The Haworth Document Delivery Service: 1-800-HAWORTH. E-mail address: <docdelivery@haworthpress.com> Website: <http://www.HaworthPress.com> © 2005 by The Haworth Press, Inc. All rights reserved.]*

KEYWORDS. Age and cancer, gay sex life, homosexuality, hormonal therapy, impotence, prostate cancer, treatment choices, treatment consequences

Bertram Schaffner, MD, is Faculty Member, Supervisor of Clinical Psychotherapy, and Chair and Director of HIV Services, William Alanson White Institute.

[Haworth co-indexing entry note]: "Prostate Cancer at Age 84." Schaffner, Bertram. Co-published simultaneously in *Journal of Gay & Lesbian Psychotherapy* (The Haworth Medical Press, an imprint of The Haworth Press, Inc.) Vol. 9, No. 1/2, 2005, pp. 131-136; and: *A Gay Man's Guide to Prostate Cancer* (ed: Gerald Perlman, and Jack Drescher) The Haworth Medical Press, an imprint of The Haworth Press, Inc., 2005, pp. 131-136. Single or multiple copies of this article are available for a fee from The Haworth Document Delivery Service [1-800-HAWORTH, 9:00 a.m. - 5:00 p.m. (EST). E-mail address: docdelivery@haworthpress.com].

http://www.haworthpress.com/web/JGLP
© 2005 by The Haworth Press, Inc. All rights reserved.
Digital Object Identifier: 10.1300/J236v09n01_11

I was diagnosed with cancer of the prostate on July 6, 1996, when I was 84 years old. I had been seeing a urologist because of difficulties in initiating urination that I had experienced since 1990, and he had been monitoring my PSA levels on a regular basis, in conjunction with needle biopsies of my prostate, which had always been negative. Despite the vigilance implied by the regular examinations, learning that I had cancer came as a shock.

I had never had a life-threatening illness before then, and my first and major concern was the question of how long I could expect to live. All that came to mind was the well-worn adage that "prostate cancer will not kill you, you will die of something else." Not yet able to obtain any information about expected longevity that I could rely on, naturally I felt under pressure to put my affairs in order, keep my will up to date, and so on. What really bothered me a lot was the fear of leaving a burden for others to take care of, and the fact that my numerous interests had resulted in a daunting accumulation of books, papers, art objects and family heirlooms of various kinds. So in addition to finding out what to do, and deciding how to cope with my diagnosis, I had the added problem of handling these concerns.

I also worried about who would provide me with companionship and care in my advanced age, and potential infirmity. At the age of 80, I began to notice that my contemporaries were dwindling due to old age and death, and I already had to make changes in my lifestyle as a result. I had been consciously developing new relationships among younger people, and keeping active in social and professional organizations. I found that in gay life, it has not always been easy for older people to make friends among younger gay people. Very often, attempts to be friendly can be misinterpreted as sexual come-ons, and rejected, which can be hard to take.

I had no previous experience or contact with others who had prostate cancer. For reasons that are very probably connected to my homosexuality, I did not feel comfortable asking questions of my gay friends and peers. I didn't like the implication that my sexual life would be over. My main concern at that time in my life was to maintain closeness to all my friends, and hopefully to establish a joint home with another gay person, and I was afraid that the revelation of my diagnosis would condemn me to aloneness for the rest of my life. I tried to table my worries about a home and to concentrate on learning about treatment.

I called the American Cancer Society, and spoke with a representative who was initially very encouraging and invited me to an interview. However, when I arrived at the Society offices and asked for services for gay people, the representative was taken aback and not only had nothing to offer, but seemed quite uncomfortable with my declaration. Needless to say, I did not return.

I inquired at Sloan-Kettering Hospital, which did have monthly self-help groups where prostate cancer patients could meet and exchange information with each other. When I got there I looked in vain for other gay cancer patients, but perhaps I was somewhat reticent in my dealings with the hospital meetings due to my experience at the American Cancer Society.

Somehow, accidentally, I heard of a gay group for men with prostate cancer that was organized privately. I got there and found the members primarily dealing with unfortunate surgical outcomes, which alarmed me, and was not particularly relevant to my situation. I attended for a little while, which gave me an opportunity at least to ventilate a bit. However, after a few weeks, a former patient of mine joined the group, and I felt that it would not be in our best interest to continue as members of the same support group.

In order to make the important decisions confronting me to ensure that I received proper medical care, I needed to gather more information about the treatments that were available at that time. Finding answers turned out not to be easy at all, and the choices quite distasteful.

Naturally, I first consulted my urologist, a straight man and surgeon. Since he might be operating on me, it was mainly important for him to find out whether I was HIV positive. Although he knew that I had been referred by a gay internist, whose practice was wholly gay, neither he nor I had ever discussed my sex life. Since the loss of ability to have an erection is usually the main concern of both gay and straight men, and the greatest danger posed by surgery for prostate cancer, it is unfortunate that we were unable to speak more frankly about sex.

He told me that my type of cancer was rated "Gleason #9," indicating a very aggressive, rapidly progressing form of the disease, and therefore in need of urgent attention. Fortunately, there was no evidence of metastasis, but very unfortunately, the tumor was no longer confined to the prostate capsule, but had already escaped into the seminal vesicles. This meant that radical surgical prostatectomy was inadvisable, because it increases the danger of metastasis.

I did not complain about ruling out a prostatectomy, as Michael Korda's (1996) discussion about his dealing with the miserable consequences of surgery had completely turned me against that route. His dramatic and heart-rending accounts of sudden urinary incontinence in public frightened me away. His long search for the "best prostate surgeon in the world" and it's unsuccessful ending, with only a bleak prospect for the future, made me rule out surgery altogether. That was 1996; today, I am told, that prostate surgery is vastly improved, as well as radiation techniques.

Then, some 9 years ago, the prevalent treatment of choice was radiation. Before I had an opportunity to explore further and to come to my own decision, I was referred to radiology. There I was told for the first time that I was to be measured for radiation of my prostate. The suddenness of the decision, and the fact that it had been made without my participation and consent, so alarmed me that I decided to consult with an oncologist, and to change my choice of hospital.

It would be too easy to blame what happened on my being gay, as if that involved a lack of respect for me, but in retrospect, I think it reflects my shyness and passivity in relation to the surgeon, and his possible difficulty in relating empathically to me. No question was ever raised about my possible concerns about future erectile dysfunction, either by him or me.

Curiously, the oncologist I consulted turned out to be a straight woman who was very empathic, already very conversant with gay patients' concerns, and who took the lead in asking me questions. However, the burden of her questions seemed to be whether I indulged in any "kinky" or dangerous sex, rather than in terms of my relationships. I suspect that she was trying to determine whether there would be any traumatic or infectious complications as a result of sexual practices. She mentioned that radiation sometimes results in injury to the rectal wall, which can be extraordinarily painful and very difficult to heal. Overall, she seemed quite sensitive to the practical aspects of gay sexuality in relation to treatment of prostate cancer, for which I was grateful.

I felt that I needed a promise from whoever was going to be my doctor that I would be given sufficient analgesic medication in case I developed intractable bone pain. As a physician, I know that there are some doctors who fear that they will be accused of causing addiction even in terminal cases with severe pain. Such doctors may think of homosexuals as more likely to request drugs for reasons of addiction. I asked my oncologist for a guarantee that she would be willing to provide me with any necessary narcotics. My oncologist was happy to assure me that she would not let me suffer.

In the light of the success that I have had with hormone therapy, it seems fortunate that she supported my fear of radiation at that particular time period. Other methods, for example, freezing, radioactive seeding, etc., were also being tried out, but there had not been enough experience with them for me to draw firm conclusions.

Having decided against radiation, I was left with the time-honored method of hormonal medical castration, with its proven effectiveness, but also its not inconsiderable consequences. It was a very difficult decision to make, but made easier by the fact that impotence had already set in by the age of 80, and I had not been sexually active for some years. In consultation with my oncologist, I decided on hormone treatment.

The deprivation of testosterone has a number of results. The predictable consequences that I would be undergoing, were complete impotence, enlargement of the breasts, hot flashes with or without drenching sweats, mild swelling of the ankles, but pronounced diminution of muscle size and strength throughout the body. There may also be more rapid osteoporosis and decrease in height. To my surprise, some of my friends began to regard me as "frail." On the other hand, my prostate has shrunk to almost nothing, is soft, and no longer palpable. Fortunately, for a long period, I had no urinary symptoms, which typically distress so many prostate patients. I slept through the night.

One aftereffect of hormone therapy demanded my attention. I anticipated and accepted the total absence of genital excitement, the tingling feeling in the penis, when I met people who attracted me, but I was at first perturbed by the absence of the ordinary psychological surge to act upon the attraction or interest. I feared that I would no longer be able to relate to people on an emotional basis, which would have left me ruinously isolated, if true.

Fortunately, I soon became aware that I had only lost the capacity to react in terms of lustful sexual interest, but that the more important capacities to feel warm, connected, and affectionate were still there in full measure, if not enhanced. It makes one think that sexual attraction can be distracting or even harmful to human relationships. I now feel much more sensitive and responsive to other human beings than I ever felt before. A wonderful compensation.

The hormonal castration has not in any way changed my sexual identity. The enlargement of the breasts, the diminution of muscle strength, and the absence of erections have not made me feel less masculine. I still feel as gay as before.

In some ways, the reduction of fear of my cancer, my increased freedom to speak my mind, and the simplification of my interpersonal relationships, have made me feel a new strength and personal integration. Despite the "castration" I really experience an increase in inner vigor, which has manifested in more writing and professional activity. I think this is attributable to less diversion of energy into the vicissitudes of romantic life.

Now at the age of 90, I am still very much enjoying the practice of psychiatry and psychoanalysis, and in addition I maintain a very active social life and cultural schedule. I do not regret the choice I made. I think it was right for me, even if it is less than optimal for people younger than myself, for whom an active sexual life is a high priority.

REFERENCE

Korda, M. (1996), *Man to Man: Surviving Prostate Cancer.* NY: Random House.

Together with Prostate Cancer

Robert P. Parkin
Howard Girven

SUMMARY. Each member of an older gay couple describes the experience of making the decision to treat their respective prostate cancers using proton beam radiation. They were in the same hospital at overlapping times. Each, in turn, discusses his reaction to treatment at Loma Linda University Medical Center and the importance of a team approach to treatment. The lack of attention to gay-related issues are addressed. The authors discuss the effect of prostate cancer, its treatment and aging on their sexual life together. *[Article copies available for a fee from The Haworth Document Delivery Service: 1-800-HAWORTH. E-mail address: <docdelivery@haworthpress.com> Website: <http://www.HaworthPress.com> © 2005 by The Haworth Press, Inc. All rights reserved.]*

KEYWORDS. Aging, brachytherapy, digital rectal exam, gay couple, Gleason score, Loma Linda University Medical Center, leuprolide acetate, oncologist, prostate cancer, proton beam radiation therapy, PSA, sildenafil, support group, team approach, urologist

BOB'S STORY

I am a seventy-six-year-old gay white man who has been living in New York City with my companion Howard for over ten years. My

Robert P. Parkin, MD, is a retired psychiatrist.
Howard Girven is a retired actor/director.

[Haworth co-indexing entry note]: "Together with Prostate Cancer." Parkin, Robert P., and Howard Girven. Co-published simultaneously in *Journal of Gay & Lesbian Psychotherapy* (The Haworth Medical Press, an imprint of The Haworth Press, Inc.) Vol. 9, No. 1/2, 2005, pp. 137-146; and: *A Gay Man's Guide to Prostate Cancer* (ed: Gerald Perlman, and Jack Drescher) The Haworth Medical Press, an imprint of The Haworth Press, Inc., 2005, pp. 137-146. Single or multiple copies of this article are available for a fee from The Haworth Document Delivery Service [1-800-HAWORTH, 9:00 a.m. - 5:00 p.m. (EST). E-mail address: docdelivery@haworthpress.com].

prostate cancer was diagnosed early in 2001 and treated with proton particle beam and conventional radiation at Loma Linda University Medical Center in California (LLUMC). Howard was diagnosed with prostate cancer about six months after I had my diagnosis. He tells his story below.

About 12 years before any definitive diagnosis of prostate cancer was made, a very small amount of PSA had been detected. My PSA gradually rose to 12 as four negative biopsies were collected. Through the years, I had discussed the treatment options available with my urologist and decided on the conservative route, to wait and see. But by 2001, my PSA had risen to 23 and cancer cells were at last found in the prostate.

Following the latest PSA and biopsy results, a more aggressive path was indicated. Having had a hemicolectomy followed by chemotherapy and radiation in 1988 for cancer of the colon, I was reluctant to have another extensive cancer treatment. Therefore, brachytherapy (radioactive seed implants) seemed the most benign procedure to follow.

My valued primary physician of many years had referred me to his urologist with whom I got on well. I trusted him in the context of what seemed to be an honest, open, and generally good relationship. However, at the time of the last biopsy, I had been quietly distressed when he told me that the resident fellow would be performing the procedure. Now, prepared to go through brachytherapy, I found myself at the oncologist's office where I was again distressed to find that the fellow's name was on the referral. With some effort, the nurse had the referral changed and reassured me that my urologist would visit after the procedure to check that the seeds had reached the intended destination. I was not reassured. He carefully explained the procedures and none of them seemed very benign. I was just beginning to explore the proton treatment at LLUMC. My urologist had heard of it and noted that some consideration had been given to it at his treatment center. He did not encourage or discourage it for me.

Loma Linda

A friend of Howard's had recently been diagnosed with prostate cancer. Having extensively explored the options for treatment, his friend decided upon the LLUMC where they specialized in proton beam radiation therapy. Howard and I reviewed the material he had amassed. We learned that the proton beam particles, split from the atom as they travel through an accelerator, can be precisely focused into the capsule of the prostate gland, sparing other tissue from damage. Concerned about my radiation history, we concluded that because the radiation problem seemed to be reduced, this was a better choice if I were fortunate enough to be accepted as a candidate for treatment at Loma Linda. With our friend's help I was able to get an evaluation appointment on the same day his was scheduled and we went there together.

My early telephone exchanges with LLUMC were friendly, informative and welcoming. At LLUMC a supportive and well functioning clinical team approach was apparent throughout the evaluation. The oncologist's nurse practitioner introduced me to the overall plan. A generous amount of time was available to speak with the oncologist who had reviewed my clinical history and reports from New York. He had also requested a recent bone scan and asked that I bring with me the slides of the cells from my latest biopsy. The session was relaxed. There was adequate time for questions. Unfortunately, the oncologist felt that the cancer had spread out of the prostate capsule into the surrounding tissue. He recommended fifteen proton beam treatments instead of the usual 40 into the prostate capsule, 25 conventional X-ray treatments as well as Lupron (leuprolide acetate) injections for at least two years. The X-rays would probably increase the risk of side effects from irradiation to the same area previously treated 12 years ago. Furthermore, Lupron can have its own side effects because it degrades testosterone. Nevertheless, following a very careful evaluation, I was accepted as an appropriate patient for their treatment protocol and I decided to be treated at Loma Linda.

I was measured for a "pod" into which patients are placed in order to maintain the consistent positioning required for the treatment. They also explained the recommended balloon (a condom inflated with water) which is placed in the rectum to aid in moving the bowel and bladder away from the proton particles during treatment. We were shown one of the treatment gantries and visited the lab where they make the wax bolus that shapes the proton beam to the precise form of the prostate gland. The beam of proton particles are split from hydrogen atoms as they pass through the accelerator at great speed and diverted to the patient by powerful computer-controlled magnets.

The coordinating social worker who introduced us to the facilities also conducted a weekly support group. I asked about attitudes toward alternative lifestyles. He stressed that although the Medical Center was under the auspices of the Seventh Day Adventists, whose commitment to healing and training of clinicians for work in underdeveloped areas was paramount, no proselytizing took place. He added that some undergraduate university students were asking for more openness about gay issues.

Various facilities of the university were available to patients: the athletic center, pool, library and housing office. The latter was very helpful in finding me a modestly priced, two-bedroom apartment a few minutes walk from the hospital. Many other residential settings are available, ranging from a motel-like campus to RV parking to luxury resort apartments.

The overall treatment experience reflected a fine example of team medicine. The nurse practitioner seemed always available when I had worrisome symptoms and appropriately involved my oncologist. A weekly meeting with the nutritionist helped me with my many gastrointestinal symptoms. The pharmacist helped me find a way to pay for my first $3000 Lupron injection.

My three weeks of 15 proton treatments were uneventful. But shortly after the conventional radiation treatments began, I experienced painful bowel movements in conjunction with constipation, diarrhea, bleeding and ulceration. Treatment with diet, cortisone suppositories, antibiotic and antiviral creams were not very helpful. My son's welcome visit, however, was very supportive. Howard arrived the following week when the symptoms became more troublesome and I involved him in the evaluation and treatment process. These stresses and hearing of Howard's diagnosis at the same time were a challenge to my independence, my wish to cope alone and my wish to be with him.

As treatment progressed, I could no longer tolerate the balloon. Tylenol (acetaminophen) with codeine helped. At one point I took a ten-day holiday from my treatment, but returned to complete it when Howard went there for his own treatment. We were together for the first week of his treatment and my last three sessions.

Support Group

I rarely attended the weekly support group until my son and Howard arrived. It seemed to be directed to the interests of straight men and their spouses. Gay issues were never recognized and my silence did not help. Jokes and humorous stories were popular and encouraged by the social worker who facilitated the meetings. I do not recall discussions about the sexual aspect of life for the individual with cancer and his spouse. Many moving stories were told about the stress patients experience as they and their families faced their cancer, finding the most appropriate and affordable treatment associated with the least damage and fewest side effects. A number of patients complained that their local urologists and urology departments had little or no knowledge of proton particle treatment. The group was very helpful in finding ways to deal with insurance carriers who were obstructionist, often making inappropriate–and what I considered illegal–decisions. For example, the insurance carriers often refused payment, stating that proton beam radiation was considered an experimental modality, and as such not covered.

However, psychological issues and sexual issues were seldom if ever addressed. I met several interesting patients and spouses. One was a poet who wrote many long, spontaneous and humorous verses about the events at Loma Linda. Patients came for treatment from all over the world. A broad, socioeconomic and professional spectrum was represented; included were a number of physicists who were knowledgeable about the mechanics and the value of proton beam radiation therapy.

Aftermath

It is now about two years since my prostate cancer treatment began (the cancer having been diagnosed six months earlier). My recovery from colon cancer had been almost complete. My PSA is negligible. Painful digital rectal examinations (DRE) were discontinued after the initial two post-treatment exams and they were negative. My gastrointestinal symptoms, associated with radiation, have gradually improved on medication, diet and increasing physical activity following a recent hip replacement.

The first three months of the planned seven months of IM Lupron treatment were unremarkable, except for their contribution to my diminished libido. But as my libido decreased, I began to experience a spontaneous period of embarrassing tearfulness and weeping, even though I was not feeling particularly depressed. I had episodes of intense and unpleasant hot flashes with associated flushing and weakness. I chose to discontinue the Lupron. About three months after treatment ended, Viagra (sildenafil) made a modest contribution to my libido and erectile function. Although I found Viagra an important resource, I discontinued it a few months later in favor of the benefits of a spontaneous sexual life.

Howard and I had been in a relationship for over eight years when, within months, we each received a diagnosis of prostate cancer. We had first met at a psychologist-led discussion group at the Gay and Lesbian Community Center in New York City and began to date shortly thereafter. We explored and found much to enjoy and nourish physically and emotionally. With homes in the city and the country, we spend more time as a couple on our own. The path we were on has gotten better over the years and has accelerated since our cancer treatments. We enjoy many things together including our sexual relationship. We like to cook, garden, and travel. Our ongoing sense of intimacy sustains us as we deal with periods of anxiety, depression, and anger. Although we were separated some of the time during our treatments, we were supportive of each other. Our lives continue to be good together.

HOWARD'S STORY

At age sixty-eight, I was diagnosed with prostate cancer in June, 2001. This happened when Bob was at the LLUMC in California being treated for the same disease. At the time of the biopsy, my PSA was 4.7, my free PSA was 9%, and my Gleason Score was 6 (3+3). My treatment stage was T1c before undergoing conformal proton beam treatment (PBT) for a localized tumor in the lower right sextant of my prostate gland. By all accounts, this is considered an early, non-aggressive and best possible situation if one has to have prostate cancer at all.

My primary physician had been urging repeat PSA's since my annual physical exam in December 2000. As I anticipated a biopsy with a positive finding, I too had been reading the material that Bob had gathered regarding the prostate, its cancer, the various treatment options and their pros and cons.

I got my biopsy report the day before going out to California to visit Bob in August. My urologist does brachytherapy and he kept saying, "It will just be a blip on your screen." When I said I had heard that sometimes a seed may end up in the bladder or neighboring organ and what did he do if that happened, he said, "I just go in and get it." He did not say how and I was too numb to ask. I took my biopsy report with me to California. I felt so depressed, I slept most of the way on the plane.

Loma Linda

The people at LLUMC were wonderful. Bob spoke to his doctor's case manager nurse who, because I had the biopsy report, diagnosis and good medical insurance coverage, proceeded to squeeze me into the intake process while I was visiting. Needless to say, the experiences of both Bob and our friend as well as seeing and talking with other patients there (who were enthusiastic to a man about the treatment and the care), I had no difficulty choosing proton beam radiation therapy.

The intake included a two-hour consultation with my oncologist and a fitting for my pod. I returned to New York to take care of affairs there, including undergoing a bone scan ordered by my urologist . Thankfully it proved to be negative. Then I returned to California where I started eight weeks of treatment.

For people with my diagnosis and staging parameters, the proton beam treatment seemed the very best way to go. That is my opinion and probably every man who has had it. As I understand from the explanations at LLUMC, the proton beam is a particle beam, which travels in only one direction. With most conventional radiations, the beam scatters in all directions (although some new developments allow some shaping of the beam) and expends most of its energy at the entry point to the body, passing through neighboring organs and the body. On the other hand, the conformal proton beam is shaped to the form of the patient's prostate and expends minimal energy at entry, rising to its greatest intensity at the target area (called the Bragg peak), killing the tumor cells. As one of their documents puts it, "Not only is the dose of radiation to normal tissue sharply reduced compared to conventional radiation therapy, but the energy of the proton beam completely dissipates within the tumor, causing no damage to normal tissues beyond the tumor."

When it comes to prostate cancer, I believe we face two major issues. The first is the threat to our lives and the second is the threat to our sexuality. Conformal proton beam treatment's rate of success is comparable to the best surgeries and conventional X-rays BUT–and it an enormous BUT–as far as I am concerned, the side effects of the two types of treatment, both during and post treatment, do not compare. And this is where proton beam radiation therapy, in my opinion, is superior to all others for those with my particular prostate cancer parameters. It is a quality of life matter.

First, the treatments themselves are simple. Proton bean radiation therapy is painless and non-invasive. During the treatment period, side effects (which vary in degree among patients, ranging from some to none) are minimal: perhaps diarrhea or constipation, some frequent or stinging urination, and fatigue–especially in the last couple weeks of treatment. However, not everyone reacts the same way. I had stinging urination in the second week and afterwards which was managed with medication. Other patients with the same diagnostic parameters and treatment plan as mine had no side effects. Until the last week, my fatigue was minimal. The staff there advises doing as much exercise as one can do. Fatigue never prevented me from taking long walks, swimming for about an hour, or both, 4-5 times a week.

Another word must be said about the atmosphere at LLUMC. The warm, caring and accessible staff, from the top down, cannot be praised enough. The hospital's mission is to heal the whole man. They believe attitude is a major part of the treatment, both theirs and the patients'. This is evident in every staff member we encountered. Every effort is made to inform the patients about proton beam radiation therapy and to understand what they are experiencing. All done in a warm, friendly way. I never felt like I was a number or that I was taking up someone's time. The experience there raised my standard of expectation for medical care.

Although I did not wave a rainbow flag about my sexuality, I did speak of Bob as my partner when talking with other patients and at the support meetings. I met no hostility but I am sure some people there may have chosen not to hear what I was saying. Nevertheless, the people I met, patients and staff, were friendly and congenial.

LLUMC has been doing prostate proton beam treatment for over 11 years, with well over 5000 patients treated. Time and again, we heard stories of patients whose doctors did not know about proton beam radiation therapy, or who said it is experimental, or that it is not effective, and who recommended that surgery or standard X-rays (or whatever treatments they themselves had to offer) was the only way to go. The patients at LLUMC have included physicians, physicists, even surgeons and urologists. These are people who know all the options and still chose PBT. As someone at my last support group meeting said, "Surgery depends on the skill of one person, the surgeon. With PBT, you have a whole team of oncologists, physicists, technicians preparing your treatment plan and then executing it. That's a lot of oversight for your treatment."

Aftermath

When I returned home after ending treatment, I experienced a good deal of fatigue and slept a great deal for about two weeks. The mild, stinging urination lasted about a week. The follow-up with my new urologist consists of PSA testing and DRE exams every six months. My last two PSA's have been excellent at 0.05. Follow-up PSA's are done for five years for monitoring as well as for developing treatment statistics.

As for the issue of sexuality, impotence can range from 30-60%, depending on the individual. My sexuality is intact, but has changed from its pre-treatment condition. The LLUMC materials say to have sexual relations during treatment if desired, with no danger to self or partner from the radiation. They also say, "the more you come in with, the more you go out with." Again this is an individual thing. I found orgasm painful after eight treatments and had some blood in my semen. My oncologist said not to worry, just remember that the prostate is in "an acute stage" and that could be expected. So I held off from having sex for a few weeks after returning home. They do not discuss the sex part much at LLUMC, I suppose on the premise that the libido may be low during treatment. However, Viagra came up frequently at the weekly support group meetings, usually jokingly but clearly in an attempt to allude to the problem of potency.

Nonetheless, I was open with the oncologist that Bob and I shared. I told him we were partners and that I wanted to know as much as he could ethically tell me about Bob's condition and our relationship. The doctor and I were comfortable discussing sex (mine, anyway). In retrospect, I realize our talks were mostly about current physical conditions and those in the immediate, post-treatment period. Longer-range sexual conditions or problems did not come up.

From the time our treatment ended late in 2001, our sexual relations have gone through and are still undergoing changes. However, they remain good. I completed treatment two months after Bob. Because of the tremendous pain I had experienced with orgasm at the beginning of treatment, I was not eager to rush back into sex. We slept together and cuddled but no stimulation was attempted for about two weeks. Bob was on Lupron at the time which caused him to experience a very diminished libido. He is a loving, considerate man. Recognizing my needs and desires, when I was ready, he offered to hold me while I masturbated. This became our practice for several weeks. I was experiencing a curious phenomenon: while easily experiencing frequent tumescence, even during treatment, I only achieved a full erection when I was with Bob. This pattern has continued.

Bob discontinued the Lupron before the planned time and has gradually regained his libido–and his potency is improving. We suspect that gay men are more fortunate than many straight men when it comes to the variety of behaviors available and used for sexual satisfaction. We have found that oral sex can be very effective and enjoyable even without a full erection. Judging from comments, albeit few, at the support meetings, oral sex was still not as common among the heterosexual couples attending as one might think in this age of frank movies and television talk shows. In any case, since recovery our sex life has become still more open and easy. Our libidos are good and we find satisfaction within our own as well as each other's body. We will adjust and adapt as time and aging impose themselves on us. We flow with the tide. And the water is fine.

My only post-treatment effects have been what I consider the normal healing process. I had understood that about six months post-treatment, some patients might experience blood in their stool and/or in their urine. Seven months after I left Loma Linda, I intermittently had blood in my stool. This was painless. It only lasted about three months and was treated with the anti-inflammatory suppository Canasa (mesalamine). As that side effect was coming to an end, I developed a bladder infection, which was easily treated with Cipro (ciprofloxacin), and may or may not have been radiation related. We looked on these as normal because the healing from radiation lasts many months and many individuals report not experiencing any after effects at all.

As Bob has said, our relationship is good and only grows better with passing time and experiences–our near simultaneous prostate cancer experience, for one. At our ages, change is to be expected and, I would hope, embraced. From our early days together, we have talked about our feelings and ourselves, starting slowly and as trust grew so did our openness. We never go to bed with a serious disagreement left unresolved. It is not a rule, rather an understanding. Well before our cancers, in acknowledgment of our eventual deaths and our status as a committed gay couple, we had prepared our wills and other legal and health care arrangements. That action and our shared brush with death have made it easier to have more open, more precise discussions about our relationship, our sexuality, our lives together, and our deaths. The threats to our lives and to our sexuality that our cancers and its treatments have forced us to face have been confronted; and we are still growing from those encounters. We consider ourselves a lucky couple.

A Gay Man and His Partner
Face His Prostate Cancer Together

Greg Higgins

SUMMARY. A middle-aged gay man describes his experience and that of his partner in facing the diagnosis and treatment of prostate cancer. The author describes his reactions to various urologists and support groups. The author offers a candid look at the sexual and psychological issues he and his partner faced when dealing with prostate cancer and the side effects of its treatment. The paper highlights the importance of patient involvement in treatment. *[Article copies available for a fee from The Haworth Document Delivery Service: 1-800-HAWORTH. E-mail address: <docdelivery@haworthpress.com> Website: <http://www.HaworthPress.com> © 2005 by The Haworth Press, Inc. All rights reserved.]*

KEYWORDS. Biopsy, gay couple, homosexuality, impotence, libido, lycopene, prostate cancer, PSA, seed implants (brachytherapy), sexuality, side effects, sildenafil, support group, urologist

THE NEWS

Like countless others, I sat across a desk from a doctor who told me that I had prostate cancer. I was fifty-five years old at the time. This

Greg Higgins, CSW, is a retired Social Worker in the New York City Department of Education.

[Haworth co-indexing entry note]: "A Gay Man and His Partner Face His Prostate Cancer Together." Higgins, Greg. Co-published simultaneously in *Journal of Gay & Lesbian Psychotherapy* (The Haworth Medical Press, an imprint of The Haworth Press, Inc.) Vol. 9, No. 1/2, 2005, pp. 147-153; and: *A Gay Man's Guide to Prostate Cancer* (ed: Gerald Perlman, and Jack Drescher) The Haworth Medical Press, an imprint of The Haworth Press, Inc., 2005, pp. 147-153. Single or multiple copies of this article are available for a fee from The Haworth Document Delivery Service [1-800-HAWORTH, 9:00 a.m. - 5:00 p.m. (EST). E-mail address: docdelivery@haworthpress.com].

http://www.haworthpress.com/web/JGLP
© 2005 by The Haworth Press, Inc. All rights reserved.
Digital Object Identifier: 10.1300/J236v09n01_13

news, which would forever alter my life, took place nearly a year after my first PSA test came back with a reading of 5.9. The value was elevated enough to merit one of those arrow indicators with the word, "high," on a piece of paper showing the results of what would otherwise have been a routine blood screening.

The first urologist to whom I was referred delayed taking any action for almost three months, despite my repeated urging that he take a biopsy. I was beginning to feel what I first took to be watchful waiting was possibly benign neglect. Perhaps I was not forceful enough.

However, both Alex, my lover of ten years, and my nephew, who had worked at Sloan-Kettering Hospital in New York City, kept insisting that I have a biopsy scheduled. Finally, after much insistence from me, the biopsy was set up for the Friday prior to Labor Day. I am a counselor in the New York City public school system; and it was my first week back to work after summer break. The timing could not have been more inconvenient. Alex and I had been looking forward to a three day weekend at the beach. But it had taken so long to schedule the biopsy, I feared trying to reschedule at that point.

My concerns escalated on the night prior to the biopsy when I received a late call from my urologist. He stated that he anticipated some equipment problems. I told him that I had waited three months for this biopsy and that I had no intention of delaying it any further. I also told him that I intended to be in his office the following morning at 11 a.m. for the scheduled procedure. I assumed that he too was looking forward to a glorious Labor Day weekend and that he only he wanted to start his getaway a day earlier.

The procedure went forward without any discussion or explanation from the urologist and with only 2 or 3 samples taken. This is, I have since learned, far fewer than the recommended number. Not surprisingly, the results were inconclusive.

My nephew urged me to find a new doctor to do another biopsy. I followed his advice and found a friendlier urologist affiliated with the New York Hospital in Queens, New York. An appropriate 10-12 samples were taken which ultimately resulted in my receiving a diagnosis of prostate cancer. Ironically, being assertive and pro-active in my own treatment unfortunately resulted in my worst fear being confirmed. What I had sought to rule out was instead ruled in. But had I waited and done nothing, the results could have been a good deal worse. I therefore cannot stress enough the importance of taking control of one's own treatment.

Upon hearing the findings, I was flooded with feelings of confusion, depression, anxiety and anger. I experienced a wide range of self re-criminating thoughts and emotions. I obsessively reviewed a ten year history of diet, exercise, and lifestyle. I blamed myself for having poor eating habits, for working too much, for not exercising enough and for anything else I could imagine. But the biggest blow was hearing my new urologist recommending the complete surgical removal of my prostate gland and seminal vesicles. Alex and I sat in the urologist's office numbed by the conclusiveness of his words. I inquired about other options, including radiation and seed implantation. He led me to believe that these options were second best. I nevertheless decided to pursue these other treatment options anyway.

Alex and I have always been open and honest with each other. I thought we had discussed almost everything regarding all the proce-dures I had gone through prior to hearing the biopsy report. But that night, after having heard the urologist's recommendation, we both went into shock and seemed to shut down. I became detached and began ru-minating about my own mortality. I was also preoccupied with the fact that I am twenty-three years older than Alex.

Alex also seemed lost in thought; but he rallied more quickly than I did. He was resolute in his conviction that the cancer had to be removed permanently. He said that he felt it had to be eradicated from my body completely, regardless of the possible side effects of incontinence and impotence. That evening, in a rare display of love and emotion, he made his feelings very clear. It touched me deeply and made me realize the depth of his love and dedication. I felt more secure for the moment, but it did not make the treatment decision any easier. Maybe the cancer could be eliminated; but I could not shake the question running through my mind like song lyrics: "Will you still love me tomorrow?" I worried about what Alex might really feel when actually faced with the reality of being with an older, incontinent and impotent man.

LOOKING FOR SUPPORT

Since that dreadful morning in the doctor's office when the prostate cancer diagnosis was confirmed, I have read many books on the subject. I pored through books about genetic causes as well as others on ancient, Far Eastern herbal cures. I also turned to other people for support. How-ever, I quickly realized how taboo the subject of prostate cancer is among men. Finally, I sought out and joined a support group for men with prostate cancer.

I recall that first meeting. There were about twenty men sitting around and participating in a group run by a female nurse with another woman from the American Cancer Society acting as co-leader. It made me wonder how comfortable women with breast cancer would feel discussing their issues in a group hosted by two men. It was obvious to me that the men were not comfortable discussing diminished sexual responses with these two women. Nor were they ready to discuss their struggles with the range of demons that plague the male psyche during the process of coming to terms with having prostate cancer. When one group member asked a question relating to dietary concerns, I encouraged him to drink plenty of tomato juice because it contains lycopene, an antioxidant that may have beneficial effects against prostate cancer. When the group leader seemed surprised by this information, I was convinced I was in the wrong place and I was out of there.

Then a friend of mine told me about a different group. It was led by a man and focused specifically on gay men with prostate cancer. I remember Alex and I entering the building with some anxiety on the night of our first meeting. However, we were told that partners were not invited that particular evening. Alex retreated to a nearby coffee shop to wait until my meeting was over.

Upon entering the room, I was immediately relieved by the presence of men, a male facilitator and no women. I thought I might finally feel comfortable enough to share my thoughts, fears and limited optimism with people who were more like me. Indeed, I immediately shared my feelings of comfort with the group. I explained how refreshing it was to find a gay men's prostate cancer support group, how glad I was to be a part of it, and how much I was looking forward to a night when partners would be invited. I wanted to hear how other couples were dealing with issues like diminished sex drive and impotence. After my enthusiastic entrance into the group, someone in the room coughed awkwardly as the facilitator gently explained, "The gay men's support group meets next week." I now laugh at the memory of that first meeting. Looking back, the entire comedy of errors parallels much of the confusion and disorientation I then felt. Nevertheless, because I wanted the support, I continued to attend the general meeting as well as the one for gay men.

At one of those meetings, I met a man who would soon become a trusted friend and advisor. He is a psychologist who had already been treated for his prostate cancer. He had opted for brachytherapy and he eventually enabled me to decide on seed implants rather than a radical prostatectomy. His manner was calm and confident. He was happy with his decision to have seed implants. I began calling him at home and he listened to the many concerns I had. He told me that he shared all my concerns about impotence, incontinence, and most especially, like me, about being a man in his late 50s concerned about keeping a long time partner many years younger than he. His partner was twelve years his junior.

He told me that research indicated both radical prostatectomy and radioactive seed implants had about the same rate of cure. It was also his reading of the research that one was more likely to retain erections after treatment with seeding as opposed to radical surgery. We each have younger lovers and we both wanted to be around for a while to enjoy the quality of life that having a younger lover provided.

Some people may be able to make treatment decisions about their prostate cancer by themselves. However, I know I needed someone I respected to push me in the direction I wanted to go, just as Alex and my nephew had pushed me to get my first biopsy and then later to change urologists. Whether it be a trusted friend, a professional or a support group, I have always found it comforting and helpful to share my feelings and thoughts with other caring people.

So with the help of my psychologist friend, my treatment moved forward. Once the procedure was over, Alex and I anticipated adjusting to our new lives and roles within the parameters defined by the treatment and its after effects.

A COUPLE'S FEARS AND CHANGES

Alex, my gentleman from El Salvador with a soft spoken manner and delightful Spanish accent, told me about what he had been experiencing since first learning of my elevated PSA level. Although he was afraid, my health and survival were always of the utmost importance to him. He was worried and concerned about me. However, it was not until after I had undergone the treatment that, then at the age of thirty-three, Alex was faced with the realities of my diminished sex drive and performance difficulties. He said, "Sometimes I get angry with you or at others for no reason, although I know what it is I am mad about. It's a little frustrating."

Both of us have often felt frustration when the two of us are out for an evening, drinking wine, and otherwise having a wonderful time. In our lives before the dreaded cancer, the evening would have ended with our making love; but now that is not always the case. Viagra (sildenafil) helps; but I think it helps Alex more than me. Although I get an erection, I seem to have a diminished sexual sensation using it.

Alex tells me that he has learned that love is stronger than sex. He masturbates a lot more often with the help of pornographic magazines, although they were not previously a part of his or our sex lives. He says he finds himself looking at other men more often than he used to, another change he attributes to my diminished sex drive.

In areas other than sex, we have also experienced shifts in the roles each of us previously played in our relationship. He used to leave everything up to me. Now Alex is more outspoken about his own opinions and desires. Our age difference seems more apparent to him now. As he accompanies me to various doctor appointments, he sees men who are usually twenty years older than him. He is a witness to men suffering from other life-threatening illnesses. He sees men who have undergone surgery and various other procedures. He sees the effects of these treatments. He has wondered what his role will become in the next ten years or so. Will he continue to be the lover, partner and friend, or will he become a nurse?

While Alex explores and wonders about his shifting roles in our relationship and the future of our sex life, I too have been dealing with some issues. I have again been thinking more about the age and cultural differences between us. We seem to many people an "unlikely couple." Our initial attraction was simply sexual, as is the case with many gay couples of our acquaintance: sex first, friendship and love later. I am concerned that I may be holding Alex back from a normal and healthy sex life. I worry about whether or not he will still be with me in the next ten years. Will I lose him to a younger, healthier man?

I too get frustrated and angry about my diminished sexual desire and sometimes lackluster performance. I sometimes get angry at Alex when I feel that I am using all my energy to make love to him because I know he wants it. Sometimes I feel that the last little drop of energy I have at the end of the day goes to him. Alex and I continue to wrestle with our issues in an arena of uncertainty.

A friend once said to me, "Isn't growing old together what it is all about?" That statement got me thinking about the twenty-three years separating me and Alex. I have thought that perhaps we will not be growing old together. After much painful discussion and philosophizing, Alex and I have decided that the only viable solution is to live in the present and enjoy what we have now.

We are currently planning to purchase an apartment in New York City. There are decisions we have to make together: What color to paint the walls, what furniture to purchase, and how to decorate. We take it one day at a time, as corny as that sounds. But we are loving each other and appreciating each other in what seems a deeper way than before as we make this journey together. Our love feels more precious.

More than twenty years ago, I sat in my psychotherapist's office, confused, conflicted and in pain. Dr. Ellis taught me that it is not the events in our life that affect us, it is how we perceive them. I learned that when an event occurs, we attach a meaning to it, a belief system, and the consequences are the feelings that derive from that belief system. I learned that I could change my belief system and in so doing change my affective reactions to the event. Instead of "catastrophizing," I could attain a certain level of acceptance. I think both Alex and I struggle to get to a level of acceptance.

Despite the differences in education, cultural backgrounds, health, and age, Alex has been there for me, often leading the way. He has a natural way of showing me that which I can easily lose sight of: That we can get there together. We love each other. And although we may not grow old together, we are certainly growing more intimate as together we struggle with the demon that is prostate cancer.

Prostate Cancer Diagnosis and Treatment of a 33-Year-Old Gay Man

Vincent M. Santillo

SUMMARY. This is a personal account of a 33-year-old gay man's discovery of his prostate cancer, its treatment, his recovery and the effect it had on his life. The paper underscores the importance of physician-patient communication, informed consent for patients, and involving the patient's partner when treating prostate cancer. In addition to dealing with incontinence and post-operative depression, the author recounts the many steps he undertook to treat erectile dysfunction as well as the difficulties that caused for him and in the relationship with his partner of twelve years. *[Article copies available for a fee from The Haworth Document Delivery Service: 1-800-HAWORTH. E-mail address: <docdelivery@haworthpress. com> Website: <http://www.HaworthPress.com> © 2005 by The Haworth Press, Inc. All rights reserved.]*

KEYWORDS. Alprostadil, cancer, depression, erectile dysfunction, gay, gay couples, homosexuality, imipramine, impotence, incontinence, informed consent, prostate, prostatectomy, sildenafil, gay relationships

Vincent M. Santillo holds a BS in Economics from the University of Pennsylvania, and an MBA from Columbia University. He is currently enrolled in the Postbaccalaureate Premedical Program at Columbia University.

[Haworth co-indexing entry note]: "Prostate Cancer Diagnosis and Treatment of a 33-Year-Old Gay Man." Santillo, Vincent M. Co-published simultaneously in *Journal of Gay & Lesbian Psychotherapy* (The Haworth Medical Press, an imprint of The Haworth Press, Inc.) Vol. 9, No. 1/2, 2005, pp. 155-171; and: *A Gay Man's Guide to Prostate Cancer* (ed: Gerald Perlman, and Jack Drescher) The Haworth Medical Press, an imprint of The Haworth Press, Inc., 2005, pp. 155-171. Single or multiple copies of this article are available for a fee from The Haworth Document Delivery Service [1-800-HAWORTH, 9:00 a.m. - 5:00 p.m. (EST). E-mail address: docdelivery@haworthpress.com].

http://www.haworthpress.com/web/JGLP
© 2005 by The Haworth Press, Inc. All rights reserved.
Digital Object Identifier: 10.1300/J236v09n01_14

155

INTRODUCTION

It all started so simply: "Your PSA is elevated and I felt a bump on the digital rectal exam (DRE). You should make an appointment to see a urologist." I had not even planned on getting a physical and I do not know why I did. Perhaps I felt some dread deep down that I could not articulate; if I did, it was not at the level of consciousness. Being resourceful, I jotted down my PSA score: 1.2. That did not seem so high, and after checking the Internet it even seemed fairly low. What I did not know, and something which does not appear anywhere on the web–perhaps the only fact that does not–is that, when they speak of a PSA level of 4.0 being a danger sign, they are talking about men in their fifties and sixties. I was 33 and invulnerable. My father had had a radical prostatectomy the year before and lightning just did not strike twice. Plus, I should not have had to deal with this until I was at least 50. My uncle had had a bad death from prostate cancer and it had killed my grandfather when he was in his eighties. I knew it was coming, but I also was sure that the technology wave that has been sweeping the world of medicine would produce a convenient remedy when my turn came to hear the words, "You have cancer." I had no inkling at all that my day to hear that was only nine weeks away.

DISCOVERY

My internist, who deserves all of my thanks and admiration for looking where others would not have thought of looking, put me at ease. He said he was "just being cautious" and that the bump "was probably a seminal vesicle" or some other benign nodule. He was right to think that. The chances that I was currently in possession of a tumor were too small to trouble myself. When I called to make the appointment with the urologist, I was not even fazed when told that his busy schedule meant I could not have an appointment for seven weeks. I went back to my summer in New York City and put the whole matter completely out of my mind.

I can honestly say that the only thing that concerned me about the appointment was that I would be embarrassed during the digital rectal exam. Things started to take a bizarre turn when I arrived in the doctor's office that morning. The waiting room was tiny, cramped and full of men older than my father. I felt like a young invader on their turf. They probably all thought I was a pharmaceutical company rep. As the room slowly emptied, there was just me and another guy who seemed to be in his fifties. He asked me if this was my first time there. I told him that it was and, after relating the details, realized that I thought my internist had been perhaps overly cautious and that I felt a little ridiculous.

I was called back by the doctor and sat across from him. After a quick introduction, I told him that my PSA was only 1.2 and that my internist said that was high. I truly thought that he would share a knowing laugh and agree that my internist was overreacting. However, his response was that my internist was right and that a man in his thirties should have a PSA of less than 1.0. That was the first sign of trouble.

We went to the examination room and he asked me to drop my trousers and bend over. The examination took just a moment and before I knew it, his demeanor changed completely. He became very business-like and told me that I needed to get cleaned up and meet him back in his office. When I sat down he said that I "had a problem" and that I would need to have a biopsy. He made a comment that since I was gay, at least fertility would not be an issue. I cannot blame him for thinking that, and I am sure that for a lot of his gay patients it is not. I just blinked at him, took my prescription for the antibiotic Cipro (ciprofloxacin) and preparatory notes on the enema I was to undergo, and was ushered out the door.

By the time I got into the street I was a basket case. I called my husband of twelve years and cried into the cell phone. It all seemed so ridiculous and absurd. We got off the phone and I found myself in front of a Catholic church. I ran up the steps and into the church. The afternoon mass was going on. I sat in the back pew and cried and prayed. Everything had been upended in my life in one 15 minute meeting. Looking back, I can chuckle at the drama of it all. But in that moment, the church, which had been a source of much pain during my coming to terms with being gay, was my only solace. I had spent seven weeks in the comfort of statistics; and now I understood how meaningless they were on an individual basis.

Life changed dramatically and almost instantly for me. That night I got home from the office and was on the phone with my mother. She said to me, "Vincent, do you think you have cancer?" For her this was not just an ordinary question. I knew that she believed that we all knew deep inside when something bad is about to happen. Like the best little boy in the world always wanting to please I told her, "I don't think I have cancer." After calling everyone who needed to know, I spent that night crying and ranting. I think that I can only remember repeating the words "absurd" and "ridiculous" over and over. The next morning I woke up early, a habit I developed immediately and of which I have not let go, and called back my mother. I told her that I had lied the night before and though I couldn't say why I thought so, I was pretty sure that I had prostate cancer. She was calm and supportive but I knew what my words meant to her.

The next week I learned all about the biopsy process. The number of technical explanations on medical websites, the many complaints on medical message boards, the vast amount of information and variety of opinions and experiences was incredible to me. Two nights before my biopsy, I even found a website that had many quotes from medical professionals debating whether or not biopsies should be taken or PSA tests given. I remember standing there screaming at my partner that here was the evidence I needed: I should not have been given a PSA test in the first place! A biopsy was ridiculous! They just wanted access to my lucrative insurance benefits! It all seems so pathetic and ludicrous now, but that night I just wanted a reason to disbelieve what was happening. I went to sleep and waited.

The biopsy itself was, in the end, uneventful. My urologist was extremely friendly and put me at ease. He even listened to me with much care when I said that I wanted to make it very clear to him that even though I was gay, that my fertility was very much an issue. He was great. He quickly apologized for an offhand comment that was not meant to dismiss me. His willingness to be open and not be defensive, to understand the anxiety I was going through, was so crucial at that moment. After all of my stress, the actual biopsy was not terribly uncomfortable. I thought the worst was over.

By the sixth day post-biopsy, my hysteria was manifest again. People always say that the worst part is not knowing. They are right. I had lost eight pounds in a week and could not take the stress anymore. I finally heard from my doctor on a Thursday evening. He said the results were back and that I had cancer. I remember saying, "I guess I am going to have to have the surgery based on my age," and he said, "It was advised." He asked me to come into his office after it closed on Friday so that we, along with my husband, could have uninterrupted time to talk about everything. My last words to him on that call were, "This is the luckiest day of my life." He agreed.

PREPARING FOR SURGERY

I had to wait six weeks for my surgery date in order for the prostate to heal from the biopsy. That seems so sad in a way; after beating it up with a biopsy needle, I would now wait until it was all better and then destroy it. Without prompting, my surgeon (he had morphed from my urologist to my surgeon after the call the day before) gave me information on donating my sperm. With so many doors closing and decisions to be made, I just could not decide on whether I would ever be a genetic father to a child. I thank God that I was at a stage in my coming out where I could discuss this with a doctor without shame.

Going to the sperm bank was a very interesting experience. The uniqueness of my situation, my relative youth and lack of wife made it slightly stranger. The documentation I had to sign discussed the disposition of the sperm in the event of my death. It presumed a female partner claiming the sperm and I had to come out to the nurse in order to ask whether my partner would have legal rights to the frozen sperm. She seemed to think that he would, but that I would need to talk with an attorney. On a more humorous note, I was asked to go into a room and told that I could watch videos or look at magazines in order to help me ejaculate. As one would expect, all of the materials were heterosexual in nature. It struck me that in a city such as New York, was it really THAT unusual for a gay man to freeze his sperm. Luckily I had brought materials of my own in order to reach climax in such a distinctly non-erotic environment (but not before taking a look at what the straight men were given to view).

A more intrusive event at the sperm bank revolved around the need for me to take a public HIV test. I was comfortable that I would test negative, but it was the first time I had taken a non-confidential test. I asked the nurse about the requirement and was told that they could not accept my sperm without a negative test result. It was unfortunate that I had to add the stress of waiting for an HIV test result, no matter how confident in the outcome, while dealing with a recent cancer diagnosis and my impending loss of fertility.

This event was repeated a week later when I went to begin donating blood for my surgery. I was told then that the blood would be tested for HIV. At that point, I knew that whatever the outcome, I had already sacrificed my privacy for my sperm and now I would have to sacrifice it again in order to donate blood for my operation. While I understand the need to do the test in both cases, I felt that any patient being given an HIV test should have some expectation of counseling in case they got a bad result. Neither the blood bank nor the sperm bank seemed particularly able to provide that counseling. I have since learned that my doctor would have received the results and then informed me himself. However, the nurses who took my blood never explained that to me.

CANCER WORLD

Another aspect of my life that changed dramatically from my diagnosis was my relationships with my friends. While a man in his fifties or sixties would at least be interacting with a peer group that was at least aware of this disease, my friends were in their early to mid-thirties. I had men ask me where the prostate was. A woman asked me if she had a prostate. While people were supportive, I felt alienated from the world. Discussions of death, cancer, infertility, incontinence and impotence were not topics to which young urban professionals naturally gravitated. One of my best friends, who had been dealing with the breast cancer of his partner's mother told me that I had "fallen into Cancer World."

Cancer World and Prostate Cancer World have their own language: mets (metastases), chemo (chemotherapy), Gleason, surgical margins, support groups, non-conformal radiation, seeds, androgens, PSA, DRE. The information was daunting. Cancer World was also incredibly supportive. At the suggestion of my surgeon, I suddenly found myself in a Gay Prostate Cancer Group. In two years I had gone from having a large family wedding with 75 people and only two other gay men in attendance to suddenly sitting at a table with a large group of gay men discussing the toughest time in our lives. It was wonderful and affirming and perhaps the best silver lining of the whole experience.

With every day as my surgery approached, my interest in my "normal" life faded into the background. My days were filled with appointments, lunches with former patients of my surgeon, and calls with gay prostate cancer survivors in Arizona. Old hobbies held no joy or interest, novels and newspapers went unread. The obsession with it was my only way to handle it. It also protected me from a world that did not understand what was happening to me. That did not want to hear about my anxiety of spending three weeks with an inserted urinary catheter. That did not want to hear my discussions about the advantages and disadvantages of pads versus diapers. I was glad to have a new group of friends to rely on, but the speed with which my previous life receded was shocking and something that I have yet to get over completely.

THE HOSPITAL

Several events at the hospital stick out in my mind. The morning of my surgery, I had been taken to a waiting area where I was instructed to change out of my clothes and to put on a gown and support hose. My surgeon was there and told me that my husband would be able to stay with me when I went into the adjacent area where my IVs and anesthesia would be initiated. The surgeon left and an orderly approached us. The orderly told my partner that he would not be able to accompany me. I told him that the surgeon had just said it was OK but the orderly said that we would not go anywhere with my husband in tow. With no alternative in that moment, I said good-bye to my husband. Too shy to kiss in an open room with an obnoxious orderly we said a quick good bye and I was off.

When we arrived in the preparation room, I was told to get up on a bed. A nice anesthesiologist came up to me with a smile and asked me how I was that morning. It was in that moment that after 33 years of worrying about what everyone else thought, whether they were comfortable, protecting them from dealing with a gay man in their midst and what that would mean, I came out of the closet AT FULL VOLUME. I started yelling at her that, "I was furious! The surgeon had said my husband could come with me and the orderly had sent him away! We had a domestic partnership agreement and medical powers of attorney and now we were being denied because we were gay!" The actual words were a lot stronger and louder. The other men in the room, some with their honored and respected wives, looked aghast. The anesthesiologist, to her credit responded immediately. She told me that the orderly was wrong and grabbed another orderly to go out into the waiting room and bring in my partner. I had always felt that I had been paranoid about the world. Yet, in that moment, one rude man had shown me that the straight world of grownups was not that different from the playground of elementary school. If you were gay you did not count. How many other men, too dignified to embarrass themselves or make a fuss, had sat alone waiting to tempt death under the surgeon's knife while their husbands sat dejected in the waiting room. It makes me angry even thinking about it. The fact that we were in New York City meant nothing. I could only imagine the horrors of dealing with an unplanned medical crisis with my husband in a less "tolerant" city.

When I got upstairs to my room after hours and hours in recovery, my entire family was there–husband, mother, father, brother, sister and sister-in-law. The looks on their faces gave away how crummy I must have looked. I however, though uncomfortable and utterly exhausted, was just so happy to have survived the surgery. The first words that my husband had said to me in recovery were that the cancer had appeared to be contained and that the surgeon had been able to spare both of my nerve bundles. This meant that I was likely to keep my erections. From that point on, I was just so happy with my decision, it was not until weeks later that I realized that my feeling of well-being might have been *slightly* affected by the amount of painkillers I was on at the time.

My four days in the hospital were fairly typical for those recovering from surgery. My whole family was there for the event and was very supportive. I was fortunate enough to be able to have a private room where my husband could stay with me 24 hours a day. It meant a lot to be able to have someone there to help me with the most basic of tasks. To go from being in the best shape of my life to the worst was an awesome experience. It is hard to imagine how difficult it was for me to even get out of bed the day after the surgery. It was all I could do to just move two feet to a recliner.

The hospital staff had their own rhythm and I enjoyed their care. My psychotherapist had made the prescient suggestion that, before the surgery, I visit the floor where I would be recuperating with a box of donuts for the nurses. When the head nurse saw me she remembered me as the man with the donuts, as I was going to be there for four or five days, I knew what a genius suggestion my therapist's had been.

I was also fortunate enough to have a surgeon who made it a point to visit me almost twice a day while I was in the hospital. These were not momentary visits, and they showed me that he was genuinely interested in my recovery and well-being. When you choose a surgeon, their hands are most important, but I learned that one's psychological recovery is also very dependent on the surgeon's ability to be encouraging of and sympathize with the patient's experience.

My relative youth compared to other people in my position was underscored one morning when a resident came into my room. He was looking at my chart while he said good morning. When he looked up, the surprise that came over his face was clear. I probably should have told him I was a young looking 60 year old. Instead, I just said, "I know. I am 33." His only response was, "How did they ever find you?" By that he meant find my cancer. I guess it is not just that it is rare for a man my age to get prostate cancer, but those of us who do probably die from it. The "why me" unfairness of cancer was always brought home to me by these experiences. Not only did I share that feeling with other patients, but I also added the "why now." I was willing to get prostate cancer as part my family heritage, but at the ripe old age of 60 when science would be able to give me a pill instead of surgery as a treatment.

RECUPERATION

On the Sunday following my Wednesday surgery I was on my way home. I was very apprehensive but I tried not to show it. I still had a urinary catheter attached to me and was not very sure on my feet. That afternoon, after we got home, I felt strong enough for the first of my many walks and my husband and I went out. I was like an old man. While I looked OK, I could not walk very fast. We walked up to the corner and back. That short jaunt left me so wiped out that we sat outside for twenty minutes while I regained my strength to return home.

The power balance in my relationship with my husband was completely upended, but I was happy to be cared for at the time. That night, as I went to bed, I placed my painkillers and a big glass of water next to the bed. I had thought of everything. At 3:30 a.m., I found myself wide awake with a fierce pain in my abdomen. It was a cold night and the comforter had ended up at my feet. Next to me, my husband slept peacefully.

The first thing I tried to do was reach for the blanket, but found that I was incapable of sitting up. I then decided to take my pills to at least solve the pain problem. It did not take me a moment to realize that if I could not sit up there would be no way for me to drink water from a glass. I was stuck like a beetle on its back, helpless, cold, pained and upset. I lay there for an hour, crying to myself. How pitiful. I was supposedly the independent one! Why should I have to wake up my husband to take a pill?! After an hour, I realized nothing was going to change my situation and I woke him up. In one minute, I was warm under the blanket and he had held me while I sat up to take the pills. I had always been so headstrong and independent, but I had to learn another way and quickly.

Two days later, my husband was going to leave me for a couple of hours to run errands. A friend of ours was going to come and spend some time with me. A couple of minutes after my husband left, my friend called to say he would not be able to come. It was a completely innocuous situation; he was an incredibly dependable friend who had been the one person whom I had relied on prior to surgery to talk to about my cancer. When I got off the phone with him, I went into a tailspin. I started crying hysterically. It completely shocked me. So many things were running through my brain: I was lonely. I was pathetic for crying. I had become dependent on others. I was a freak. How could I care that someone could not visit? For three hours I cried without a break. I had already changed so much and I did not like it. I was vulnerable. I just could not put on my game face and when my husband returned I cried even harder.

My gregarious life was gone for the time being. It was not just the fact that I did not feel up to seeing people. I had no shame about having a catheter bag and physically I could have spent time with friends. It was that I did not know what to say. I had always used humor to deal with difficult situations and I admitted to myself that I had not been able to find the funny side of cancer, yet. Without that perspective, I felt unable to discuss how pathetic I felt. My husband and I withdrew for weeks. We took walks and rested.

Finally the day came when the catheter was to be removed. I had read all of the literature that said that the younger and more continent a man was prior to a radical prostatectomy, the more quickly the incontinence would be gone. Perhaps it would even be gone with removal of the catheter. Another young man I had met with prostate cancer had told me he was dry within two days and prophesied that my experience would be the same. It was with some excitement that I had it taken out. I was able to stop my stream for the urologist and everything looked good. I could not figure out how to use the Depends pads so I just opted for the diaper I had brought with me. By the time I had stepped into the street, however, I discovered what I was in for. With every step, the urine squirted out of me. No matter how I clenched, it just ran. My husband and I had been planning to go to get some breakfast in a diner that morning, one of my first outings. With things as they were, he said he would understand if I would prefer to just go home. My response was, "No." This was the hand I was dealt and no one at the diner would know what was happening. So why should I go and hide in my room? Sometimes it helps to be shameless. This was not my fault and I was not going to feel bad about it right then.

One good thing about the catheter being out was that I could finally take my penis for a dry run, so to speak. It felt strange but good. There was not even a hint of an erection, but where there is a will there is a way. When I had my first post-op orgasm it struck me how strange it was to shoot blanks. My next thought was, "Thank heavens!" It is one thing to lose your erections, quite another to lose the pleasure of an orgasm. At the time, I appreciated what I had and held a lot of optimism that where orgasms were erections would soon follow.

One other milestone of my recovery was my first solo foray out of the apartment. It is hard to explain how nice it was to put on some headphones and walk the three blocks to the pharmacy to pick up my prescriptions. My partner had been apprehensive, but I had my phone with me and felt strong enough to do it. It took me all of twenty minutes but brought me a lot of joy. I was back in the world and independent, at least for a short while.

My thirty-fourth birthday was six weeks after my surgery and, after first thinking I did not want to see anyone, I decided to plan a dinner for ten friends at a local Italian restaurant. I was off painkillers at that point so I would finally be able to have a little bit to drink. It was a terrific night. I felt like my old self. I was laughing and joking. Making fun of diapers, catheters and hospitals. The next day when my best friend called me to say that it was wonderful to have the old Vincent back, I knew that I had completely fooled everyone. It seemed they were ready to move on. They did not want to deal with me being sick anymore. It was my gift to them.

The next week I had my second post-op PSA test and got my first prescriptions for impotence and incontinence. The medicine for the incontinence was an antidepressant (imipramine) that had a side effect of making it difficult for patients to urinate. Just the right side effect for me. It worked like a charm on the incontinence, but, even at the low dose I was taking, I realized why Prozac (fluoxetine) had been such a hit. I could not focus and constantly found myself in a fugue state. Three days after I started taking the drug, I stopped. The cure seemed to me worse than the disease.

It took another two months for my incontinence to end. It went like this for several weeks–I would have a setback, get depressed, do more Kegels (an exercise for tightening sphincter muscles), have a good day and feel better. One day I forgot to put a pad in my underwear and headed off to work. By the end of the day, I realized that I had dripped only once and from that point on the pads were gone. Finally, instead of thinking about prostate cancer every time I leaked or went to the bathroom I could go without thinking about it for extended periods. It was only when I felt sexual that it came back to the forefront of my mind.

SEXUALITY AND DEPRESSION

As I alluded to above, I had also been given a prescription for Viagra (sildenafil). When the pharmacist handed me my little pill container with four pills I said, "There must be a mistake, my prescription was for twelve pills." The pharmacist said my plan only covered four per month. As my urologist had told me to take one a week at night when I slept to stimulate nocturnal erections, I was floored. Four pills left me none for sex! I told her to give me the other eight and I would pay for them myself. At almost $10 per pill, I do not know what made me angrier–the insurance company, which did not feel a man my age deserved to have sex or the fact that I was reduced to begging for my erections from the female pharmacist.

The next morning, my curiosity got the better of me and I popped a Viagra. Forty-five minutes later, my head started feeling stuffed as the blood rushed to it and my vision developed a distinctive blue tint. I started to masturbate and was saddened to see that not much was happening. I had a slight engorgement so at least my penis did not look as pathetic as it had. But it was not hard enough to really grab or do anything. Just then my husband woke up and walked into the room. With a big smile I showed him what was going on. This slight physical improvement gave me a lot of confidence that my future was bright. Unfortunately, two months later I realized that the slight engorgement was all that I got from Viagra. It was a bust! I was one of the many men for whom Viagra did not work.

Two weeks later, when I had stopped sleeping at night and was constantly anxious, I knew that I needed professional help. My surgeon had warned me to watch for a possible depression two to three months post-op and it arrived right on time. I had never really understood what depression was. To me, it had always been a matter of cheering myself up, putting on some upbeat music and getting on with things. This time was different. It started with me getting up at 3 a.m. and not going back to sleep. I did not feel particularly anxious, but found myself spending night after night in cancer chat rooms on the Internet talking to people in Australia where it was daytime. I once again stopped calling friends. My birthday had unfortunately been an anomaly. I had been able to convince everyone that I was well, but I did not have the strength anymore. After an argument with my husband, about nothing particularly memorable, I found myself unable to calm my anxiety. While I never truly considered suicide, the thoughts flashed through my mind. It was at that exact moment that my phone rang and my internist was on the other end of the line. I put on my happy voice and had a quick chat. I mentioned that I had been anxious and not sleeping and he gave me the name of a doctor to see about it. I look back now and am thankful that I did not let myself suffer any longer than necessary.

By this point, my positive outlook was waning. I now felt myself cured of cancer. But I was very angry at being incontinent, a difficult thing for anyone to handle and anathema to a control freak like me. I was absolutely furious with my penis for being completely dead. The quality of life issues, which had been in the background for the first couple of months of my recovery, were taking center stage. My sex life with my husband had quieted down. He was unable to bring me to orgasm, which, while possible, was difficult to do with a flaccid penis. He tried not to let me know, but I knew that it must not have been much of a turn-on to be in bed with me. We quietly let the time between trying sex lengthen as we each dealt with our feelings on the matter in isolation.

At my three-month check-up, I mentioned to my urologist my disappointment with Viagra. He suggested that I try Caverject (alprostadil). I already knew what that was, but naively asked him what it entailed. If there is one thing that will make most men cross their legs and run from the room, it is the idea of sticking a needle into their penis. I said that I was not ready for that and would give myself more time. He said to give him a call if I changed my mind.

Two weeks later, I called his office and made the appointment. Fear usually makes me react with strength and I was determined to not give up on my erections. Even to have just one would be of huge psychological benefit. I went in for the appointment. The first shot is given by the urologist to target the dose. It was fairly painless and I found myself looking away as it was done. Ten minutes later, I had my first true erection in three months. It felt great! I then realized that it also was going to be around for a couple of hours. I called work to let them know I would not be coming back in and headed home. One side effect of the injected drug is an aching pain around the entire groin area. By the time I got home, the pain was significant. I just sat in a chair waiting for it to abate. While I was happy with the Caverject's result, I also realized how much I truly missed the functioning body I had before the surgery. I knew deep inside that I had another battle ahead of me, that while relatively less dangerous than dealing with my cancer, was just as dark and filled with fear and anxiety. I had not thought about it before, but now that the cancer was behind me, my impotence moved front and center.

THE LONG-HAUL

My husband, by this time, was beginning to fray at the edges. While I had been in acute crisis mode, he had been supporting me and taking care of me. Now that some degree of independence and health had returned, he started to slip into a very natural post-traumatic stress induced depression. He had a harder time hiding his sadness every time we made love. One morning after we had tried to make love (I had not picked up my prescription for Caverject yet) I lay down next to him and asked him what was wrong. He told me that he could not stand the pills, the injections, all of it. It was too "weird." I promised him it would not go on forever and went to shower. I know that his comments were a reflection of his own anger with my cancer, but I could not stop myself from taking it personally. I was furious. This was not my fault. He had promised to love me "in sickness and in health." Wasn't this sickness? Was I going to end up alone and a freak? To top things off, I felt I could not let him know how upset I was because then he would just completely shut me out. We both smiled at each other, but we had lost the ability to communicate on the topic for the time being.

Two weeks later, I came home with my Caverject prescription and we decided to give it a try. It was not the best sexual experience of my life, but it was the most memorable. It was so incredibly ordinary that I almost found myself choking up throughout. I did not want to break the mood by acknowledging how wonderful it was to feel normal in bed together so I did not say anything to him. I really thought we had found a solution that would get me through the two years it might take until I regained natural erectile function.

The next weekend we decided to try again. This time it was a disaster. By the time we got into bed, I was fully erect. I could feel his detachment from what we were doing. He himself did not at all seem to be aroused. After lying in bed for 30 minutes without really getting anywhere, I got up and stormed out of the room. An hour later, as we sat and talked about what had happened, he admitted that it all felt "so mechanical." What was I to do? If I could not get hard he was unhappy. If I used the only thing that got me hard he was unhappy. It was perhaps the toughest time in our twelve years together. This was the one crisis with which I could not help him. I was trying to pretend that the shots were fine, they were normal, and they were just as good. Inside I was terrified that this was going to be my life for the next fifty years.

On the morning of my operation's sixth-month anniversary, I called my internist. He reiterated that it would take six months to two years to regain function. He tried to focus me on the range of times, but I just wanted someone to tell me everything was going to work out. He did his best, but I am still watching the clock. Two years seemed like not much time before my surgery. Now that it is my potential "prison sentence," assuming it does not turn into a "life sentence," the time seems to crawl. My husband and I love each other, of that I am convinced. However, we still cannot seem to be able to get on the same page or discuss the topic with any resolution. It is hard to be objective when someone is upset with you at a situation caused by your own body and over which you have no control.

SILVER LININGS

Several months after my surgery, I was watching a television interview with an oncologist and she said something which really struck me, "The thing about cancer patients is that getting a diagnosis like this can sometimes bring an appreciation of life to people. They want to live every day to the fullest, to let the little things slide, to reevaluate their path. That is something as an oncologist that I can help them to appreciate." I am no stranger to that sentiment. I had been reconsidering my profession prior to the cancer and the diagnosis really moved that along. My previous attitude of "I'll figure out what I really want to do and do that when I am 45" seemed foolish.

Several years ago, I had gotten an application to a post-baccalaureate premedical program (a stepping stone to medical school for those who have non-pre-med undergraduate histories). I had decided not to pursue it because it "was too late," "I had made my career decision," I was comfortable and afraid of change. Now I felt fearless. Why not look into it? Why not consider it? My intense experience with the medical profession over the last several months had really shown me what a difference someone could make in another's life. Most important, it was not just the physicians' technical skills that made it bearable, even though they were excellent. Instead, it was their ability to communicate clearly with me and to understand that, in my case, the more information they could provide the better. My surgeon even jokingly referred to my "intellectual arrogance" for trying to become an expert on prostate cancer in six weeks.

Almost nine months to the day after my cancer surgery, I will begin my classes. It is an adventure. Balancing school at night with a daytime career is going to be grueling. I have already started working in an Emergency Room to get some more direct exposure to what I may expect. It is a terrific way to spend Friday nights. My internist and surgeon, who provided me with so much guidance through my cancer treatment, have taken on additional roles–being both cheerleaders and detractors. Challenging me to really know what I am getting myself into, grilling me on my motives, while providing me the encouragement to explore it to its ends.

Should I go forward with a career in medicine, I think this experience can only help to make me a better doctor. To understand what it means to be told bad news and to fight your way through that. Should I decide at some point that my desire to help is satisfied by volunteering, then that too will be OK. At least I will have taken advantage of a willingness to reevaluate my life and to make a conscious decision based on who I am today and not who I was when I went to school to study finance as an 18 year old.

Someone recently said to me that, "I bet if you could you would wish away the last year." My response was "No way!" While I would have preferred to be educated in a less dramatic way, I would never trade what I had learned about myself in the last several months for anything in the world. The cancer was probably written in my genes from the moment I was conceived, it was supposed to happen, it is part of my story. How can I regret that?

CONCLUSION

At this point, just past six months post-RRP, I am still going to keep my hopes up. I have much to be thankful for: my cancer seems to be gone, my strength and vitality have returned, I have learned a tremendous amount about myself, and I am continent. However, that small germ of fear that my sexual function will not ever improve haunts me. And I worry that my anxiety and fear about it will grow with each passing day. I only hope that either I recover or, much like with the cancer diagnosis, I find some strength and coping mechanisms that I have not yet tapped into that will get me through whatever life throws at me. Just this morning, my assistant put an article in my inbox that she had photocopied from a major business publication. It pertained to neural grafts, which were being done during prostatectomies to help those whose nerves could not be spared. The final paragraph mentions a patient who had a nerve graft and was waking up four months later with erections. His final statement was, "How many women would want a guy with a broken ding-a-ling?" For a 62-year old like him, that seemed a tough situation. For me it seemed like a nightmare. Needless to say, I had a bad day after reading that.

Epilogue

As this article nears publication, I felt some update to my story was in order. It has now been more than two years since my surgery. My PSA's have all been undetectable and according to my surgeon, I am cured. In addition, I am continent and able to achieve erection unaided though sometimes I use a prescription drug to help it last longer. The last two years have held both positive and negative surprises. But on the whole, I am healed. My husband and I are working through our issues, and we have settled into a new life together that is far stronger for having been so tested. Perhaps, equally as challenging has been the 250+ hours spent in an Emergency Room and lots of late night classes. I am six months away from applying to medical school and look forward to applying what I learned from my experience as a patient to a future medical practice.

Glossary

Gerald Perlman, PhD

ADENOCARCINOMA: A form of cancer that develops from malignant abnormality in the cells lining a glandular organ; almost all prostate cancers are of this variety.

ADJUVANT THERAPY: Treatment used in addition to the main treatment, such as radiation therapy and hormonal therapy which are often used as adjuvant treatments following a radical prostatectomy.

ANDROGEN: Any male sex hormone. The major one being testosterone.

ANTIANDROGENS: Drugs that block or interfere with the body's ability to use androgens at the cellular receptor sites. Antiandrogens used to treat prostate cancer include the brand names Eulexin, Casodex, and Nilandron.

ANTICHOLINERGIC: A drug that may block the parasympathetic nerves; such as blocking the bladder and genitalia. May be used to treat urinary incontinence, among other conditions.

BENIGN PROSTATIC HYPERPLASIA (BPH): Non-cancerous enlargement of the prostate that may restrict urine flow.

Gerald Perlman is Former Director of Psychology Internship Training, Manhattan Psychiatric Center.

[Haworth co-indexing entry note]: "Glossary." Perlman, Gerald. Co-published simultaneously in *Journal of Gay & Lesbian Psychotherapy* (The Haworth Medical Press, an imprint of The Haworth Press, Inc.) Vol. 9, No. 1/2, 2005, pp. 173-178; and: *A Gay Man's Guide to Prostate Cancer* (ed: Gerald Perlman, and Jack Drescher) The Haworth Medical Press, an imprint of The Haworth Press, Inc., 2005, pp. 173-178. Single or multiple copies of this article are available for a fee from The Haworth Document Delivery Service [1-800-HAWORTH, 9:00 a.m. - 5:00 p.m. (EST). E-mail address: docdelivery@haworthpress.com].

BIOPSY: A procedure in which the physician places a narrow needle through the wall of the rectum into the prostate in order to obtain samples of tissue to ascertain if cancer is present. This is done with the guidance of ultrasound.

BRACHYTHERAPY: A form of radiation therapy in which radioactive seeds are implanted in order to kill surrounding tissue. Also called interstitial radiation therapy or *SEED IMPLANTATION (SI).*

CAPSULE: The fibrous outer lining of cells around an organ such as the prostate.

CARCINOMA: A form of cancer that originates in tissues which line or cover a particular organ.

CATHETER (URINARY): A thin, flexible tube through which fluids enter or leave the body. It is common for prostate cancer patients to have a transurethral catheter (Foley) in order to drain urine for a period of time after certain treatments.

CAVERJET: A brand name of alprostadil which is a drug used to treat erectile dysfunction (*ED*). It is injected directly into the penis; it produces an erection by relaxing the trabecular smooth muscle and by dilating the cavernosal arteries localized in the penis. See *MUSE.*

COMBINED HORMONAL TREATMENT (CHT): The blocking of the production of androgen (prostate testosterone) through surgical or chemical castration plus the use of antiandrogen hormone therapy. Also called total hormonal ablation, total androgen blockade, or total androgen ablation.

CONFORMAL RADIATION THERAPY (CRT): Planning and delivery techniques designed to focus radiation on the areas of the prostate and surrounding tissue that need treatment while protecting areas which do not need treatment. 3-D CONFORMAL therapy (3-D CRT) is a sophisticated form of this method.

CRYOSURGERY: Freezing of the prostate transperineally in order to kill the tissue, including cancerous tissue, by using liquid nitrogen probes guided by transrectal ultrasound imaging of the prostate. Also called *CRYOABLATION.*

DIGITAL RECTAL EXAMINATION (DRE): The physician's use of a lubricated, gloved finger inserted into the rectum in order to feel for abnormalities of the prostate and rectum.

DOWNSIZING: The use of hormonal or other treatment forms to reduce the volume of prostate cancer in and/or around the prostate prior to other curative treatment.

DYSURIA: Painful or burning urination.

EXTERNAL BEAM RADIATION (EBRT): A form of radiation therapy in which the radiation is delivered by a machine focused on the area affected by the cancer. Also called *EXTERNAL RADIATION THERAPY.*

FLOMAX (tamsulosin): A drug used to relax the prostate and bladder neck to improve urine flow.

FREE-PSA: This indicates how much PSA circulates unbound in the blood and how much is bound together with other blood proteins; i.e., the percentage of free-PSA to total-PSA. A low percent of free-PSA (25% or less) suggests that a prostate cancer is more likely to be present. It is a useful screening device when PSA values are above normal but less than 10. Also called *PSA-II.*

GLEASON SCORE: A method of classifying prostate cancer cells on a scale from 2 to 10. The higher the number, the more undifferentiated the cells, the faster the cancer is likely to grow. A ranking of 1-5 is assigned to the two most predominant patterns of differentiation present in the tissue sample examined. These numbers are added together to yield a total Gleason Score. Scores of 2-4 indicate well differentiated cells; 5-6 indicate tumors with cells beginning to scatter; and scores of 7-10 indicate poorly differentiated cells.

HORMONE THERAPY: The use of medication or surgery to interfere with hormone production or action. Because prostate cancer is usually dependent on male hormones to grow, hormonal therapy is used to block or lower testosterone.

HIGH DOSE RADIATION (HDR): The temporary implanting of radioactive seeds into the prostate, followed by external beam radiation (*EBRT*).

IMPOTENCE: The inability to have or to maintain an erection. Erectile dysfunction (*ED*).

INTENSITY MODULATED RADIATION THERAPY (IMRT): A computer generated program that pinpoints the cancer for radiation treatment.

INCONTINENCE: The loss of urinary control.

KEGEL EXERCISES: Exercises designed to improve the strength of the muscles controlling urination.

LUTEINIZING HORMONE RELEASING HORMONE (LHRH): A chemical that blocks the production of testosterone by the testes which may be used as part of hormone therapy of prostate cancer. Lupron and Zoladex are common brand names.

LYCOPENE: An antioxidant found in tomatoes, raspberries and watermelon; laboratory studies have indicated that it may have a beneficial effect against prostate cancer. Also available as a dietary supplement.

MUSE: A brand name for a form of alprostadil in the form of a suppository inserted into the urethra for erectile dysfunction. See *CAVERJET.*

NADIR: The lowest point reached, for example, in a series of PSA values following radiation.

NERVE SPARING: A term used to describe a type of prostatectomy in which the surgeon saves the nerves that affect sexual functioning.

NOCTURIA: The need to urinate frequently at night.

ONCOLOGIST: A physician specializing in the treatment of cancer.

ORCHIECTOMY: The surgical removal of the testicles; castration.

PARTIN TABLES: Tables that use PSA, Gleason score, and clinical stage of prostate cancer to predict the likelihood of organ confinement, as well as capsule, seminal-vesicle, and lymph-node involvement.

PARTIN II TABLES: Tables that use PSA growth rate after prostatectomy to distinguish local recurrence from distant metastasis.

PC SPES: The brand name for a dietary supplement that is used to lower PSA in prostate cancer; it is no longer available. *PC Plus* appears to be a new generation of this herbal supplement. See *SAW PALMETTO.*

PERINEAL PROSTATECTOMY: An operation to remove the prostate gland via an incision made between the anus and the scrotum (the *PERINEUM*).

PROSTATIC INTRAEPITHELIAL NEOPLASIA (PIN): A pathologically identifiable condition thought to be a possible precursor of prostate cancer. Also known as *DYSPLASIA.*

PROSTATE: The walnut sized gland in the male reproductive system that surrounds the urethra and is immediately below the bladder. Its primary function is to supply fluid for semen to transport sperm during ejaculation.

PROSTATECTOMY: The surgical removal of part or all of the prostate gland.

PROSTATE-SPECIFIC ANTIGEN (PSA): A protein secreted by the prostate gland. It is used to detect potential problems in the prostate and to follow the progress of prostate cancer therapy. Elevated levels may indicate an abnormal condition which may be malignant or benign.

PROSTATITIS: Inflammation of the prostate. It is not cancer.

PROTON BEAM THERAPY (PBT): A form of radiation that uses protons to treat cancer tumors; the proton beam is focused on the cancer site. Protons are subparticles of an atom that are absorbed by the tumor. Also called *PROTON BEAM RADIATION.*

PSA VELOCITY (PSAV): The rate at which PSA values increase. A higher PSAV indicates a greater likelihood of cancer being present.

QUALITY OF LIFE (QOL): An evaluation of health status relative to a patient's age, expectations, and physical and mental capacities.

RADIATION ONCOLOGIST: A physician specializing in the treatment of cancers with the use of various types of radiation.

RADIATION THERAPY (RT): The use of radiation to destroy malignant cells and tissues.

RADICAL PROSTATECTOMY (RP): Surgery to remove the entire prostate gland, the seminal vesicles and nearby tissue.

RETROPUBIC PROSTATECTOMY: The surgical removal of the prostate through a vertical incision in the abdomen.

SAW PALMETTO: One of the eight herbs that comprise *PC SPES*. It decreases the bioavailability of testosterone in laboratory studies.

STAGE: A term used to define the size and extent of a cancer.

TRANSPERINEAL: Through the perineum.

TRANSRECTAL: Through the rectum.

TRANSURETHRAL RESECTION OF THE PROSTATE (TURP): A surgical procedure to remove prostate tissue obstructing the urethra and thus urine flow.

WATCHFUL WAITING (WW): The active observation and regular monitoring of a man with prostate cancer without actual treatment. Also called *EXPECTANT MANAGEMENT*.

RESOURCES

American Cancer Society (1999), *Prostate Cancer Treatment Guidelines for Patients.*
American Foundation for Urologic Diseases (1998), *Prostate Cancer Resource Guide.*
Winick, L. (2000), *The Reference Guide for Prostate Cancer.* Jericho, NY: Health Education Literary Publisher.

Index

BOOK ORDER FORM!

Order a copy of this book with this form or online at:
http://www.haworthpress.com/store/product.asp?sku=5473

A Gay Man's Guide to Prostate Cancer

____ in softbound at $19.95 ISBN-13: 978-156023-553-8. ISBN-10: 1-56023-553-5.
____ in hardbound at $29.95 ISBN-13: 978-1-56023-552-1. ISBN-10: 1-56023-552-7.

COST OF BOOKS _____

POSTAGE & HANDLING _____
US: $4.00 for first book & $1.50
for each additional book.
Outside US: $5.00 for first book
& $2.00 for each additional book.

SUBTOTAL _____
In Canada: add 7% GST. _____

STATE TAX _____
CA, IL, IN, MN, NJ, NY, OH, PA & SD residents
please add appropriate local sales tax.

FINAL TOTAL _____
If paying in Canadian funds, convert
using the current exchange rate,
UNESCO coupons welcome.

❏ **BILL ME LATER:**
Bill-me option is good on US/Canada/
Mexico orders only; not good to jobbers,
wholesalers, or subscription agencies.

❏ **Signature** _____

❏ **Payment Enclosed: $** _____

❏ **PLEASE CHARGE TO MY CREDIT CARD:**
❏ Visa ❏ MasterCard ❏ AmEx ❏ Discover
❏ Diner's Club ❏ Eurocard ❏ JCB

Account # _____

Exp Date _____

Signature _____
(Prices in US dollars and subject to change without notice.)

PLEASE PRINT ALL INFORMATION OR ATTACH YOUR BUSINESS CARD

Name	
Address	
City	State/Province	Zip/Postal Code
Country	
Tel	Fax
E-Mail	

May we use your e-mail address for confirmations and other types of information? ❏ Yes ❏ No We appreciate receiving
your e-mail address. Haworth would like to e-mail special discount offers to you, as a preferred customer.
We will never share, rent, or exchange your e-mail address. We regard such actions as an invasion of your privacy.

Order From Your **Local Bookstore** or Directly From
The Haworth Press, Inc. 10 Alice Street, Binghamton, New York 13904-1580 • USA
Call Our toll-free number (1-800-429-6784) / Outside US/Canada: (607) 722-5857
Fax: 1-800-895-0582 / Outside US/Canada: (607) 771-0012
E-mail your order to us: orders@haworthpress.com

For orders outside US and Canada, you may wish to order through your local
sales representative, distributor, or bookseller.
For information, see http://haworthpress.com/distributors

(Discounts are available for individual orders in US and Canada only, not booksellers/distributors.)

Please photocopy this form for your personal use.
www.HaworthPress.com

BOF04

WITHDRAWN